# Pain Relief without Drugs

## A Self-Help Guide for Chronic Pain and Trauma

### JAN SADLER

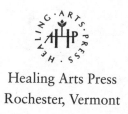

Healing Arts Press
Rochester, Vermont

Healing Arts Press
One Park Street
Rochester, Vermont 05767
www.HealingArtsPress.com

Healing Arts Press is a division of Inner Traditions International

Originally published in the United Kingdom in 1997 by Element Books under the title
  *Natural Pain Relief: A Practical Handbook for Self-Help*
Second edition published in the United Kingdom in 2001 by The C. W. Daniel
  Company, Ltd.
This third edition published in 2007 in the United States by Healing Arts Press under
  the title *Pain Relief without Drugs*

*Note to the reader: This book is intended as an informational guide. The remedies,
approaches, and techniques described herein are meant to supplement, and not to be a
substitute for, professional medical care or treatment. They should not be used to treat a
serious ailment without prior consultation with a qualified health care professional.*

**Library of Congress Cataloging-in-Publication Data**
Sadler, Jan.
  Pain relief without drugs : a self-help guide for chronic pain and trauma / Jan Sadler.
  — 3rd ed.
      p. cm.
  Originally published: Natural pain relief. Shaftesbury, Dorset : Element, 1997.
  Summary: "A practical, effective, and inspiring guidebook for dealing with chronic
pain" —Provided by publisher.
  Includes bibliographical references and index.
  ISBN-13: 978-1-59477-151-4 (pbk.)
  ISBN-10: 1-59477-151-0 (pbk.)
  1. Chronic pain—Alternative treatment. I. Sadler, Jan. Natural pain relief. II. Title.
  RB127.S23 2007
  616'.0472—dc22
                                                                      2006029560

Printed and bound in the United States by Lake Book Manufacturing

10  9  8  7  6  5  4  3  2  1

Text design and layout by Priscilla Baker
This book was typeset in Sabon

*For Colin,*
*my constant source of love and encouragement*

# Contents

# Acknowledgments

I am deeply grateful to all those who have contributed in any way to the making of this book.

An enormous thank-you to: the late professor Patrick Wall, for reading the manuscript and most kindly writing the foreword; Dr. Chris Wells, Consultant in Pain Relief, Liverpool, for his supportive comments and his practical suggestions and ideas at the editing stage; Dr. Brian Roet, for reading the manuscript and for his encouraging words.

A special thank-you to all my family and friends for their love, support, and encouragement. And, finally, my gratitude to all the people in pain who have written to me over the years.

# Foreword

I applaud Jan Sadler for writing this book and urge her readers to cherish and relish it as they would a good new friend.

There are some pains that physicians and surgeons can take away, and they are welcome to them. I don't think that readers of this book have pains of this type or they would have no reason to be even this far into the book. One pain of this sort is the dreadful stabbing pain in the face called trigeminal neuralgia. Most people with this pain respond wonderfully to tablets, and if they do not, simple, safe, highly effective neurosurgery stops the pain. For this pain doctors and surgeons can act in their traditional authoritarian way. They can "take away" the pain as a welcome act of theft with little need to involve the victim. How nice it would be if all pain treatment was like that: the equivalent of taking a splinter from the hand. Many doctors and some patients act as though it were this way. The doctor issues a prescription and orders, "Take these three times a day and come back and see me in a month." The passive, obedient, "good" patient announces, "I am *under* the doctor's orders."

In the real world, there are far more common pains, such as arthritis, where this attitude not only is not common but also leads to anger and frustration for both doctor and patient. It is true that tablets and sometimes surgery can lead to considerable improvement, but they do not wipe out the pain in the dramatic way the first type of pain can be treated.

Many years ago I witnessed treatment in hospitals in China. I was delighted and astonished by the relaxed and cooperative atmosphere. As a foreigner, I often had difficulty in distinguishing staff from patients.

I was repeatedly told, "We recruit the patient to be a member of his own treatment team." That is what all doctors should do and what all patients should demand. The patient must be informed and involved so that the team can achieve the best possible results. Jan Sadler's book helps in this cooperative effort.

Last, there are some types of pain, such as fibromyalgia, where the greatest experts in the world do not yet understand their origin and no medicine or surgery can specifically wipe them out. In some ways these are the worst types of pain because they isolate the victim. Some old-fashioned doctors and even friends and relatives tell the victim "There is nothing wrong with you" because there is no detectable cause for their pain. No one can find the "splinter" at the site of the pain. The victims are abandoned and sad. Now comes Jan Sadler, who believes in the reality of these people's pain and suffering. She has been through it herself. She shows a path, which requires bravery, in which the patient adopts some of the responsibility to explore and aid his or her own condition.

For those of us who work professionally on the problems of pain, we must redouble our efforts to discover the origin of pains, particularly those of unknown cause and those treated with ineffective therapies. For all of us, in or out of pain, we should applaud those who struggle to understand their personal pains and to bring them under the forms of control this book describes.

PROFESSOR PATRICK D. WALL, DOCTOR OF MEDICINE, FELLOW OF THE
ROYAL SOCIETY, FELLOW OF THE ROYAL COLLEGE OF PHYSICIANS

Patrick Wall (1925–2001) was a renowned neuroscientist whose research into the mechanisms of pain led to several new forms of pain treatment, including the TENS (transcutaneous electrical nerve stimulation) machine, which interferes with pain pathways from the spine to the brain. He was professor of anatomy at University College London from 1967 to 1990 and then emeritus professor based at St. Thomas's Hospital. Early in his career he spent time in the United States, teaching at Yale, the University of Chicago, Harvard, and MIT. He co-edited the first textbook on the subject of pain, *Textbook of Pain,* and founded *Pain,* the premier journal of the field. He left behind a legacy of associates and students to continue his pioneering research.

# Introduction

*The natural healing force within each one of us is the*
*greatest force in getting well.*

HIPPOCRATES

It doesn't matter where the pain is, how intense it is, how long you may have had it, or what caused it: you will find relief from that pain in this book. You, like me, already have the capacity to reduce your own pain. You have hidden powers and strengths deep inside yourself that are the means of energizing your own natural healing powers. With the practical activities in this book you can release and maximize your full healing and pain-relieving potential.

After a back injury and operation, I found that drug therapy alone was unsatisfactory in dealing with the pain and so I began to develop my own personal coping strategies. On my journey I made many wonderful discoveries about my own natural inner powers to reduce pain and discomfort, to make changes and to regain control of my life. My success led me to make programs for others on how to cope not only with pain, but also with how it affects many aspects of our lives. Eventually I put this book together for all those who are looking for a way to help themselves. I live with pain's challenges daily, and so the book is written from my personal knowledge and experience of techniques that work for me and for thousands of other people, and they will work for you too. When I was first struggling with pain, there was little support available; this is the book I would have liked to have kept by me.

The way you experience your pain is closely linked in a unique way with your own personal reactions. Your personal reactions are within your own power to influence and change. The techniques in this book will show you how to make the changes you desire. The book has a structured but flexible approach and is packed with ideas that will enable you to have a new dynamic sense of being in charge of your situation and will help you to reduce and live more peacefully with your pain. As well as helping you to lessen your physical discomfort, this book will also show you how to foster your self-esteem and how to lead a fuller, more enjoyable life.

Work at your own pace with the techniques in the book, and please don't tackle too much when you start. You may feel like taking on some of the ideas now and some perhaps in a few weeks, months, or even in a year or so. Remember, you don't have to do it all at once. One step at a time, that's all we can do. Be gentle in your approach and use the techniques with an attitude of respect and kindness toward yourself. Enjoy the activities: they are written in your best interests, for your good and your benefit. Do listen to the recording that accompanies this book. As well as adding another dimension to your experience, it will enhance your understanding and enjoyment of the relaxation and visualization exercises.

The techniques in this book are meant not necessarily to replace any treatment, conventional or alternative, you may be having, but to be used alongside it as a complement. Even if you are having treatment of some kind, *you* are still the only one with the power to cope with the pain and the effect it may have on your life. With these techniques, you can learn to use your personal power to work *with* the treatment and *with* the pain.

## WHERE TO BEGIN

You can begin by listening to the CD or you can look through the book first; it doesn't matter, as one enhances the other. The book is set out in units, each one devoted to a particular aspect of natural pain relief. The units are self-contained, giving full details of helpful, easy-to-understand, stimulating and practical techniques. Some of the activities are very short and quick to do and some require more time and thought.

There's no need to sit down and read the book through, as one would a novel; this is a book to dip into, in any order. So, before you decide where you would like to begin, browse through the book to get some idea of the contents. If you are new to natural pain relief, a good place to start is with Unit 1, about relaxation, and then work through the book from there. If you have picked up this book when you have a pain flare-up, Unit 9 deals with these and you may prefer to start there. Those of you with some experience in self-help may find that some of the units contain techniques that are familiar to you and in which you may be skilled already, but there is still sure to be something new within the units for you to try. Best of all, start wherever you feel you would *like* to start. The book is merely a guide to all the wonderful techniques available; take from it what you need, when you need it.

Remember this: no matter what your situation, there is *always* something you can do to reduce the pain and improve your lifestyle. Let the book be a friend and a guide to you. You are no longer alone; join the many others who are taking this same journey with you and me.

# UNIT 1
■
# The Power of
# Deep Relaxation

## CONTENTS

# The Power of
# Deep Relaxation

We have within us a natural inner power with the ability to give us deep peace, tranquillity, and relief from pain. We can release these wonderful sensations by learning a special breathing and relaxation technique. This is one of your most important resources to help reduce your pain and encourage self-healing. This inner power has always been there and always will be there, available for you to call upon whenever you feel the need. Learning how to use your breath to foster deep relaxation can improve your life dramatically.

It is possible to obtain almost immediate freedom from pain and discomfort with deep relaxation. The relief from pain may last for the duration of the relaxation session or you may benefit from lower pain levels over a longer period of time. The more you practice, the better and more effective the relaxation and relief will become. If you can give yourself the time to relax deeply once or preferably twice a day, you will feel calmer and more in control of your situation and be well on the road toward a more comfortable, pain-reduced life.

Remember, we can *all* do this—you don't have to be a special sort of person. This inner power is with us when we are born, but it tends to lie forgotten or unused within us. Learning how to relax and allow peaceful and calm feelings to come to the surface was the very first way I started to help myself. My first experience of relaxation was a revelation to me. It was just wonderful to find such quiet stillness and freedom from pain.

Now, you may think you already know how to relax or that you are relaxed as you watch TV, read, or rest quietly, but what is meant here by relaxation is quite different. The deep relaxation that can release your inner powers of healing and pain relief is at a different level from that achieved by just sitting or lying down. You are seeking to allow all your muscles to relax and all the internal rhythms and organs of your body to slow down. Tight and tense muscles not only cause pain but also prevent your healing processes from working efficiently. Even if you think you are relaxed, it's quite normal for your body to be full of hidden tensions. For instance, as you read this, check around your body. Try the following body check now.

## MUSCLE TENSION CHECK

*Is your jaw tight? . . .*
*Is your forehead furrowed? . . .*
*Are your hands gripping the book unnecessarily hard? . . .*
*Are your legs twined around each other? . . .*
*Are your toes curled up?*

You may have released some muscle tension during the above body check but you are, most probably, quite unaware of many other muscle tensions that still exist in various parts of your body. This is because we become so used to holding ourselves in a particular way that we fail to notice the tensions anymore. We didn't start off like this; these tensions have built up over the years. We have become out of touch with our own bodies; thus, we erect barriers that prevent nature's own healing powers from helping us as effectively as they might. Through relaxation we can allow the release of many or all of these tensions and start to feel much better, even finding we have no pain at all for a while. Relaxation is cumulative, so if you add on relaxation and calmness throughout the day, you will soon notice the difference in your life.

You may notice I have been talking about "allowing" relaxation to happen. It is something we cannot *make* happen; trying hard to relax merely adds tension. In the same way, we cannot *make* ourselves go to sleep; we have to let go and allow sleep to creep over us by itself. To achieve deep relaxation, we have to give ourselves permission to let go and give freedom to our inner healing.

## OUR BREATH—THE KEY TO RELAXATION

The more understanding we have of what happens during relaxation, the more we will appreciate the importance of our breath, which is the key to deep, peaceful, pain-relieving relaxation. Our breath is always there, available to us with this amazing, almost magical facility. During a full relaxation session, our breathing deepens and slows down. This allows muscles to relax and blood flow to increase, nourishing all parts of our body and encouraging our internal systems to slow down. We begin to feel heavy, warm, and comfortable and we may even become unaware of our body altogether. The slow, deep breathing during relaxation promotes a feeling of general well-being, it reduces our heart rate, and, best of all, endorphins, the body's own natural painkillers, are released into our bloodstream. Our mind slows down and we feel very peaceful and calm. All these effects stem from the way we breathe during relaxation.

We all tend to take our breathing for granted, not noticing anything very much about it. Many of us, especially when in pain, use an inefficient type of breathing, whereas correctly used, our breath can become our most powerful ally; and so, first of all, *how* are you breathing?

### Breathing Check

*Check your breathing right now. Put one hand on your chest and*
*another between the bottom of your rib cage and your abdomen.*
*Just let your hands rest there for a few minutes.*
*Then notice which hand moves more.*

The lower hand is the one you would hope to find moving more for normal, quiet breathing. This is called diaphragmatic breathing.

Our diaphragm is a large, dome-shaped muscle that is attached all around the lower part of our rib cage. The diaphragm is like a floor to our rib cage, filling the space between our chest and the organs in our abdomen. When we breathe in, the diaphragm moves downward, pushing out the abdomen; the whole of our rib cage expands and our ribs move sideways and outward at both the front and the back of our chest. When we breathe out, the diaphragm returns upward, allowing the abdomen to fall, and the old, used air is expelled. This is the most healthy and efficient way for us to breathe. If, instead of using diaphragmatic breathing, we habitually use the neck, shoulder, or top of the chest muscles, we breathe quickly, shallowly, and inefficiently and can even make ourselves feel tense and unwell.

Deeper, diaphragmatic breathing has the effects of relaxing all our muscles and of allowing the oxygen taken in on the in breath to be used more effectively, to feed and regenerate all the cells of our body. On the out breath, waste products from the cells are removed, ridding our body of impurities. In this way, our whole body is nourished by our breathing. Diaphragmatic breathing is also essential for the optimum function of many other systems of our body. Thus, you can see that by allowing deeper, slower diaphragmatic breathing, we nurture ourselves in many ways.

An excellent start toward natural pain relief is to practice diaphragmatic breathing every day. An exercise similar to the one below can also be found on the CD accompanying this book.

### Breathing Practice

1. *Lie down on the floor or on your bed with a thin pillow under your head and, if this is comfortable for you, another, larger pillow under your knees. This last pillow is often particularly helpful if you have a back problem. Make sure your clothing is loose, especially around your rib cage, waist, and abdomen. Spend a few moments allowing your body to soften and relax down into the surface beneath you.*

2. *Become aware of your breathing and just observe it for a moment as your breath flows in and out. Breathe through your nose, as this filters and warms the air. Let your breathing be slow and steady. Notice the in-and-out movement of your rib cage and abdomen. Don't do anything; just watch what happens as you breathe. You may notice your ribs moving at the side and may also feel the expansion of your back against the floor or bed.*

3. *Place your hands between the lower part of your ribs and your*

*abdomen and you will feel the rise and fall of your breath. As you breathe in, the area rises and as you breathe out, it falls. No other part of your body needs to move, so check that your upper chest and shoulders are still.*

4. *Continue watching this deep diaphragmatic breathing for as long as you like, at least five minutes. Be sure not to force your breathing mechanism in any way; this is a process that takes place quietly and naturally. You will gradually become more and more relaxed, allowing body processes to function normally and smoothly; endorphins will flow and the healing process will be enhanced.*

Practice like this as often as you can each day, perhaps four or five times. Once you have practiced lying down in this way a few times, practice Steps 2, 3, and 4 when you are sitting and standing. When sitting, be sure to maintain an upright and poised posture. If you slump, there is no room in your body for the expansion of your rib cage and diaphragm. Diaphragmatic breathing will soon become your normal way of breathing for much of the day. Once the pattern of breathing is established, you may want to continue with the practice anyway, because it is so relaxing and pleasurable. You may find this breathing practice so effective that you use it as your main form of relaxation.

## BASIC RELAXATION METHOD—THE BODY SCAN

Relaxation is central to natural pain relief. The following Body Scan makes an excellent basic relaxation practice. Use it once or twice a day to bring peace, tranquillity, and comfort to your body and mind. With the Body Scan you are able to be in touch with your body in a deeply nourishing way.

When you use the Body Scan, you lie down, or sit, where you can be comfortable and then take your mind around your body, spending a minute or two with each part, getting to know it. You feel and "sense" each part in minute detail, allowing it to soften, sink down, and relax onto the surface beneath you, letting any tension flow away from you. You will feel relaxation spread in waves as your muscles let go and lengthen. You don't have to "do" anything: just allow it to happen—and it will.

Each out breath carries away tension and cleanses your body, each in breath brings peace and a renewal of vigor and health; your natural healing process is under way.

As you go through the Body Scan, you'll find that you are feeling either more and more heavy and warm or very light and warm, as though you are floating. As you complete the session, you will feel as though your whole body has melted away. You will be conscious only of your breathing, which will become very light and completely effortless, as though your body doesn't exist. It is a wonderful sensation, bringing stillness, peace, and freedom from pain. The peaceful, calm feelings can remain with you for some time afterward.

I like to do the Body Scan lying down on my back, on the floor, with my head on a few paperback books or a thin cushion to give it a little support. I bend my knees, pointing them toward the ceiling, with my feet a little way apart, flat on the floor. I rest my hands on my abdomen, not letting them touch each other. You can lie on your bed if that is easier for you than lying on the floor, and lie with your legs and your arms straight if you prefer. If you would rather sit, make sure you are really comfortable with your back, head, and arms well supported, your hands apart, not touching each other, your legs uncrossed, and your feet on the floor.

### How to Practice the Body Scan
Listen to the Body Scan on the CD that accompanies this book. Or you may choose to record the following script on tape or have it read slowly to you, leaving plenty of pauses, especially where you see the dots. If you choose to listen to the CD, it will still be helpful to read through the exercise below.

1. *Find a quiet place and take off your shoes and loosen any tight clothing. Lie down where you can be comfortable and warm. Make sure you won't be disturbed for fifteen to twenty minutes.*

    *Become aware of your breathing and for a moment or two just notice the gentle rise and fall of your chest and abdomen as you breathe in and out. . . . Let your eyes close if you'd like.*

    *On the next out breath (the in breath will take care of itself), let your breath out through your mouth with a slight sigh, with just a hint of a smile about your face. The smile will help to relax your whole face. . . . The sigh will allow your breathing to become deeper and more effective. . . . Breathe in through your nose.*

*On the next out breath, imagine the sigh going down from the top of your head to the soles of your feet. . . . Feel the relief as you let the air go and allow all the tension to drain away. . . .*

*Your whole body feels more and more comfortable and at ease. . . . Feel it begin to sink down into the surface beneath you. . . .*

2. *As you move in your mind through your body, allow plenty of time with each part to gain full benefit from the attention and to allow relaxation of the muscles: say, for the duration of three in and out breaths for each body part.*

*Start by becoming aware of your head resting down into the surface beneath you and allow your neck to be soft and free. Your neck is an especially important area to keep free and relaxed. It's rather like a gateway; if we open the gate, we allow relaxation to spread from our neck throughout our body. Travel slowly in your mind around your head, letting your head sink down into the support beneath it. . . .*

*Move your awareness to your face and feel your forehead widen and relax as you bring your attention to it. . . . Notice the muscles letting go. . . . Take your attention to your eyes; let them soften and relax. . . . Let all the tiny muscles around your mouth relax; allow yourself a gentle half-smile. . . . Your jaw is relaxing and even your teeth and gums are relaxing. . . . Let your tongue lie gently in the bottom of your mouth. . . .*

*Return to your neck and allow it to soften and relax some more . . . at the front, the sides, and the back. . . .*

3. *Continue in this same way all around your body, allowing each part to soften and let go, spending about three breathing cycles in each area. Travel slowly on from your neck down your back . . . spending time with your lower back. . . . Return to your neck and relax that area again . . . then go to your shoulders . . . then down both arms . . . to your hands . . . and on to your fingertips. . . . Move on to your pelvis and abdomen . . . and then go down both legs at the*

*same time, spending time with your thighs . . . knees . . . calves . . . ankles . . . and finally go to your feet and toes. . . . Allow each part to soften, relax, and let go of tension. . . . Occasionally your mind may start to wander; if it does, return to paying attention to your breathing for a while and then continue with the Body Scan.*

4. *Complete the relaxation by returning to your neck, head, and face. Your neck is soft and free. . . . Your head is heavy and relaxed. . . . Your forehead feels cool . . . and as smooth as silk. . . . Your eyes are soft and at ease . . . all the tiny muscles around your eyes are letting go. . . . Your cheeks are soft and peaceful. . . . Your jaw is relaxed. . . . Your teeth are slightly apart. . . . Your lips are barely touching . . . and your tongue lies softly in the bottom of your mouth. . . . Your whole face is smooth, serene, and tranquil. . . .*

5. *You have brought peaceful relaxation to all of your body. . . . You may now feel very heavy and warm or you may feel very light, as though your body is floating and full of space. . . . Your body is at peace and your mind has slowed down. . . . Let thoughts pass through without getting involved with them; just watch them from moment to moment as they arise and float away again. . . . They are nothing to do with you, you are the onlooker, the watcher of thoughts only. . . . If you find you are getting hooked up with following your thoughts again, return your attention to your breath. . . . Remain like this for as long as you can, enjoying the sensation of having totally "let go."*

6. *To complete the session: when you are ready, become aware of the room and stretch out your arms and legs. . . . Take the feelings of peacefulness and calmness back with you as you gently start to move again. . . . Know you can regain these feelings at any time. . . . The peace and relaxation are always there for you.*

## Ways to Extend the Relaxation

Try one of the following ideas if you would like to extend the relaxation.

1. *Breathe relaxation and warmth in to and out through any part of your body needing your special attention. Feel as though your breath is coming in and going out from that area, as though there is a special breathing place there. Imagine you are breathing warmth, relaxation,*

*and healing right into the area that needs healing. Imagine the area being softened, soothed, and calmed. Keep breathing in and out like this for as long as you like, ending the session as in the Body Scan.*

2. *Say to yourself, inside your head, a word or two to reinforce the relaxation in your mind, such as,*

> *"Peace . . ."*
> *or "Be still . . ."*
> *or "Relax . . . [on in breath] . . . release . . . [on out breath]"*

*Continue to breathe gently in and out, using the words on each in or out breath for as long as you like, completing your session as at the end of the Body Scan relaxation (page 13).*

### Practicing the Relaxation

For the most successful results, practice the Body Scan relaxation once, preferably twice, every day, for at least a month. After that, you may alternate the Body Scan with any other relaxation or meditation method if you'd like. To achieve this daily practice, you need to make a promise to yourself to set aside twenty minutes or so, actually *making* the time for relaxation. Now, this may seem easy, but it's amazing how many excuses we can find for not taking this time out! Don't underrate your mind's ability to sabotage your good intentions, even though you know inside yourself that it will be to your benefit. Be firm with yourself and make it an absolute priority to keep your relaxation appointment.

When you begin to let go at the start of the relaxation process, as your body settles, you may become aware of a little localized twitching in your body or eyelids. This will soon pass and is best ignored. As you relax, occasionally you may also become more aware of your thoughts and feelings, perhaps feelings of sadness at your pain. Again, be glad of the opportunity to release this negativity because once you allow it to surface, you become free of it. Just quietly continue with the Body Scan or with diaphragmatic breathing and you will soon progress to deeper relaxation, where thoughts and feelings become quiet.

Soon you will find such benefit from the Body Scan relaxation that you will look forward to your session and will do it because you enjoy it and find it so pain-relieving and refreshing. These days I make sure I don't skip my Body Scan because I appreciate the great value of getting in touch with myself in this way.

The Body Scan is also extremely good to use last thing at night to help you ease into deep, peaceful sleep, or for those times when you wake up and are unable to drop back off to sleep. Take yourself through the Body Scan and you can be sure you will be asleep before you have completed it.

If you live in a busy household, do tell your family and friends you need to set aside about twenty minutes each day when you won't be disturbed. Explain that it is part of a new program to help you control your pain. They will understand and appreciate it when they begin to see the beneficial results.

Training yourself to use diaphragmatic breathing and the Body Scan gives you the means of relaxing deeply at any time without having to use a recorded version, which, although useful, may be inconvenient—for example, at night, in company, or when you are away from home.

## MINI-RELAXERS

In addition to using a full-length relaxation every day, it is extremely helpful to have "mini-relaxations" throughout the day. You will be able to maintain the benefit from your full relaxation by learning how to spot tension buildup and by knowing how to release it.

You can use your knowledge about breathing and relaxation in various ways that take only a minute or so. Mini-Relaxers are suitable for any situation and any time of day, whether you are alone or with others, in a car, standing in line, in a room full of people—all without anyone noticing. Imagine, your own portable pain reducer . . . free and always available.

Read through the Mini-Relaxers, and *try* them. It is through *experiencing* and practicing them that you gain benefit. The techniques are quick and effective, so use one or the other often during the day. When taking these short relaxing breaks, you feel more in touch with your real self and come away refreshed and energized.

### The Tension Spotter

This is a method of spotting and releasing tension around your body.

*Stop what you're doing and be still. You can even say* STOP *to yourself, quietly but firmly, either inside your head or out loud. This will surprise your mind and leave a moment's clear space, allowing you to change what you are doing; this is especially useful if you notice negative thoughts flying around inside your head or if you notice pain building up in your body.*

*When you have stopped what you are doing, scan around your body in your mind to see if you can find tension anywhere. Check your feet, legs, back, shoulders, arms, hands, neck, and face. You may find that just by placing your attention on, say, your shoulders, the muscles will start to release and let go: not by actually moving the part you have your attention upon, just by* thinking *about it. Let each area become softer and release as you move, in your mind, around your body. Finally, soften your lips—they should hardly be touching—and let your tongue lie gently in the bottom of your mouth.*

*If you have difficulty in noticing any tension, it may be useful to tighten the area first, tense it, and really feel the contracted muscles—and then let it go. Try this to see if it helps.*

Follow the Tension Spotter with this Portable Pain Reducer or use either on its own.

### The Portable Pain Reducer

*Bring your mind to your breathing; don't do* anything, *don't try to alter it, just follow the breath as it flows in through your nose and down to your lungs, follow the rising and falling of your lower ribs and abdomen, follow the breath back out again through your nose. Concentrate more on your out breath. See if you can bring a slight smile to your lips as you breathe out. Close your eyes briefly if you want to. Notice how your breathing becomes slower and deeper.*

*You can repeat this for five or six breaths. Use this short diaphragmatic breathing practice at any time during the day or night when you become aware that your body needs extra caring and nurturing.*

*If there is time, continue by saying to yourself inside your head:*

*"I allow myself to relax."*
*"My feet are heavy, they are sinking into the ground."*
*"My shoulders are relaxed and heavy, they are dropping down."*
*"I am peaceful . . . [breathe in] and calm . . . [breathe out]."*

*Repeat each sentence three times, if time allows. You may find that just one of these statements becomes the most effective for you and is your favorite. If so, just use that one. As always, adapt everything to suit you.*

A Mini-Relaxer will allow you to become calmer, reduce any pain, and enable you to carry on with renewed energy. Use it as soon as you start to become aware of increased pain; it will help to stop it from building up. As you gain experience, you will become more in tune with your body's needs and have a greater awareness of when to stop for a mini-relaxation.

## REMEMBERING TO REMEMBER

Although Mini-Relaxers are easy to do, the hard part is *remembering* to do them. You could try some of these ideas until you are accustomed to stopping regularly during the day to give yourself some care and attention.

- *Post small notices around your home, in the car, or at work.*
- *Set a timer for every half hour or hour.*
- *Stick unobtrusive small circles at eye level in strategic places around your home; these will mean "relax" to you.*
- *Place special objects around your home or your work environment that mean "relax" to you—for example, a certain vase, ornament, or even your watch. When your eye falls upon it, stop and relax.*

The natural healing powers you release by using the breathing and relaxation techniques in this unit are the key to successful pain relief, so practice, practice, and practice some more until you can regain comfort and tranquillity at will. *Always remember that this natural inner power has always been there for you and that it always will be there. NOW you know how to release it and use it.*

## ACTION GUIDELINES

1. Tell your family and friends about your need to set aside this quiet time each day that will help you control your pain.
2. Start with the diaphragmatic Breathing Practice; this is the basis for all relaxation and natural pain relief. Practice a few times every day for at least a month and then once or twice a week as a "reminder."
3. A few days after starting the Breathing Practice, introduce the Body Scan relaxation. Make time for one, preferably two, twenty-minute sessions for yourself every day. Remember, you have to *make* the time. Promise yourself that, no matter what, you will keep to these sessions. These are times just for you and are of vital importance to you.
4. Take a few minutes now and then throughout the day to stop what you are doing, whether you think you need to or not—especially if you are very busy or have a flare-up of pain. Use the time for a Mini-Relaxer.
5. Treat yourself to simply watching the clouds, listening to music, appreciating some flowers or a beautiful painting—do anything that will enable you to let go and stand back from life for a short while at intervals during the day. You will be greatly refreshed and able to progress with your day more easily.
6. Use the CD that accompanies this book and build a collection of relaxation recordings. The reference section at the end of the book includes information on ordering additional recordings.
7. *Practice, practice, practice.*

# UNIT 2

■

# What Are You Telling Yourself?

**CONTENTS**

# What Are You Telling Yourself?

*Life is shaped by the mind. We become what we think.*

BUDDHA

We all know about the benefits of positive thinking and of having a positive attitude toward life. A positive attitude influences the way we feel; we feel confident, enthusiastic, happy, joyful, and in control of our lives. It is of particular importance to you and me because it is well proven that our thoughts directly affect the functioning of our bodies; our thoughts translate immediately into physical or emotional reality. No sooner do thoughts enter our minds than changes occur in our bodies or emotions; it is as instantaneous as switching on a light. Think how wonderful this knowledge is. It means we can actually have some influence on our bodies and emotions and can make a positive contribution to reducing our pain and healing ourselves.

We all have a tremendous healing force within our bodies. Our bodies have a natural self-righting or healing mechanism that strives continuously to heal and repair any damaged part. All the individual cells in our bodies are already doing their best both to heal us and to lower our pain levels by producing endorphins, our own natural painkiller. With the encouragement of a positive attitude, they can do even better.

# HOW THOUGHTS AFFECT YOUR EMOTIONAL AND PHYSICAL BEING

By carrying out the following two experiments, you will prove for yourself that your thoughts, your emotions, and your body are inextricably linked. First of all, test how your thoughts can change your emotional state.

## Test Your Thoughts and Feelings

Your emotions are the products of your thoughts. How you feel at this very moment is as a result of your previous thoughts. To illustrate how this works, spend a few moments doing the following experiment. Do try this personal research for yourself; it is quite illuminating.

### Step 1

1. *Take a few moments to notice how you are feeling right now. What are your thoughts? What are your emotions? How does your body feel?*

2. *Now, for the sake of this experiment only, spend a few moments thinking about your pain and the ways in which it has restricted your life.*

3. *Notice how you are feeling now. What are your thoughts? What are your emotions? How does your body feel?*

4. *Clear your mind of this negativity by imagining that those thoughts and feelings are leaves on the ground; you have a broom and are sweeping them vigorously away.*
   *Carry on immediately with Step 2.*

### Step 2

5. *Cast your mind back to a time or situation where you were happy or remember an event you found funny, when you remember laughing. Shut your eyes if it helps to get a clear picture. Make the memory as sharp and bright as you can; see if you can remember colors, sounds, what you were wearing, and what other people were doing. Really live the moment again. Spend a short while thinking about this event.*

6. *Notice how you are feeling now. What are your thoughts? What are your emotions? How does your body feel?*

From this experiment, you can see how different thoughts produced different feelings. The input of positive thoughts produced feelings of happiness and pleasure; you may even have found yourself smiling as you remembered the event.

### Test Your Muscles

Now, try this muscle test for yourself. It will show you quite vividly how closely our thoughts and physical bodies are interlinked. As before, this needs to be experienced, so take a moment for this dramatic experiment.

1. *For this experiment you will need a piece of paper; writing paper will be fine. Use your dominant hand—that is, the hand you write with. Hold the piece of paper firmly between your thumb and your third finger. Now, hold the other end of the paper with the index finger and the thumb of your other hand. Test the strength of your grip by trying to pull the piece of paper out from between your thumb and third finger. You will find this very difficult to do. (Please don't overdo the pressure on the paper or you may make your third finger sore.)*

2. *Next, for the sake of this experiment, you should now deliberately introduce some negative thoughts. With the paper held as before, between your thumb and third finger, tell yourself you are a weak and powerless person, a victim of pain. Now try again to pull out the paper with the thumb and forefinger of your other hand. You will find the paper slips out quite easily. Your muscles will have immediately become weaker because of your negative thoughts. Now, very quickly, in order to rid yourself of the negative thoughts, blow all the thoughts away, as though you were blowing the seeds from a fluffy dandelion seed head; see the thoughts floating harmlessly away, like little parachutes. At the same time, shake your hands to rid them of any unwanted vibrations.*

3. *Last, grip the paper again in the same way and this time treat yourself to lots of positive thoughts. Praise yourself and tell yourself how wonderful you are, that you are strong and invincible and in charge of your life. Now try to pull out the paper. You will find that this time your muscles are full of strength and the paper cannot be easily*

*removed. The positive thoughts have given instant strength to your body.*

## BUILDING A POSITIVE ATTITUDE

These two experiments will have given you some idea of the power of our thoughts to affect both our bodies and our feelings. Imagine the healing that can take place with the right thoughts. Yes, we can encourage self-healing, with all the cells of our bodies functioning more efficiently and producing those wonderful pain-reducing endorphins for us. With positive, strengthening thoughts we can also choose to enhance the way we feel, encouraging a more serene and uplifted spirit within ourselves.

I appreciate that we are often told to "be positive" and I understand how you may feel when hearing this remark in the face of your pain. You may have tired of being told to "be positive," perhaps thinking, "It's easy for 'them' to say because 'they' don't have the pain" or "Anyone with this pain would be fed up." This sort of negative attitude is always easy to justify by saying we are only being "realistic" about our position. However, it is not the situation itself that is causing us to think these and other negative thoughts. A situation may be a *challenge,* but no situation is "bad" in itself. It is our attitude toward the situation and our interpretation of it that is important. *We may not be able to change the situation, but we can change the way we view it.* We may not be able to wish away the pain but we can change how we feel about it.

We can learn to befriend the part of our body that is troubling us, respect it, and be patient with it. We can learn how to help it to function more efficiently by not forcing it to do what it now finds difficult. We can learn how to relax, to pace our activities, and to take advantage of all the many other wonderful ways in which we can use our own natural powers to help ourselves. We can learn how to keep our thoughts positive and supportive. We can grow to understand that we are more than our pain and have deeper parts of our being that can be content and happy despite our physical difficulties. Being positive means *focusing* on the positive aspects of life and on what we can do to help ourselves. *Remember: positive thoughts are not a luxury—they are essential to our well-being.*

## THE THINKER IN YOUR MIND

This new positive attitude sounds like quite a major way in which to change yourself, but it is actually quite simple. Your attitude, and this includes your attitude to your pain, comes from the thoughts you think. Having a positive attitude does not mean, of course, that you never have unhappy, angry, fearful, or disapproving thoughts in your mind. It is perfectly normal and acceptable for any and all kinds of thoughts to come into your mind.

However, your attitude to life, and to your pain, will not be in your best interests if you constantly allow unhappy thoughts to dominate in your mind. Remember, the thought comes before the emotion. It is your interpretation of life, and of the pain, that causes either a discouraging attitude or a supporting one.

You can't control the thoughts coming to your mind but you can choose which of those thoughts you follow. Your thoughts are not a power in charge of you; the power lies behind the thoughts with you, the real *you*, the thinker of the thoughts.

As you saw with the experiments, your thoughts influence your physical and emotional states. As you discovered, you change the thought and you change the feeling; you change the thought and you change the way your body functions. It is as simple as that. If you change your thoughts, you can change your attitude. And, yes, you *can* change your thoughts—you can stop a negative thought and deliberately replace it with a more life-enhancing thought. Although you may not always realize it, you do not have to spend time chasing limiting thoughts through your mind. You do actually have a choice in the way you handle your thoughts.

By understanding that you are the thinker in your mind, the inner wisdom behind the thoughts, you can accept the power to believe you can change your attitude. However long you may have been thinking in a certain way, it is *never* too late to change to a new way. You always have the freedom to choose your thoughts.

To understand this power, imagine for a moment that your thoughts, as they arise in your mind from moment to moment, are like the names of the various foods available on the menu in a restaurant. When you come to choose your meal, you appreciate that you don't have to eat all of the dishes on offer but you *select* from the menu the foods that appeal to you. You scan the whole menu, then discard or ignore those options you don't like or want and then select the dishes you *do* like. We don't have to choose the curry if we'd rather have the salad.

Thoughts are similar. Just because you *think* a particular thought does not mean it is important, that you have to take any notice of it or concentrate on it. You can choose to either follow a thought or let it drift away from you.

Yes, you can choose not to linger with downbeat thoughts. As you read this book, many thoughts will run through your mind. Although we are often unaware of it, our minds produce a variety of thoughts all the time. Your thoughts may range, for example, from thoughts about what you're having for dinner, what you have to do next, that it's someone's birthday next week, how soft and furry your cat feels when she nuzzles you, right through to worry thoughts, thoughts about the pain or perhaps about whether the ideas in this book are really going to help you. All these and any other thoughts are perfectly natural and normal for all of us.

You may notice that some of the thoughts in all this mental chatter are positive, some neutral, and some negative. What you need to realize is that none of them are "bad," they are just thoughts. Developing a positive attitude does not mean you never have negative thoughts. What it means is that it's your responsibility as to what you *do* about them.

As the thoughts, whatever they are, come to your mind (to the attention of the thinker, that is), you may notice that you mostly pay them little attention, you dismiss them after you have scanned them. For instance, you don't necessarily spend time going over and over the thoughts about your dinner or your friend's birthday; your attention soon goes on to another thought or interest. You can do the same with any discouraging thoughts. You can learn to let this type of thought float through your mind without it affecting you. You can learn to refuse to pay attention to negative, blocking thoughts, choosing instead to focus your mind on more constructive, upbeat thoughts.

This needs practice, so you may want to consider yourself "in training" for a while until it becomes more like second nature to concentrate on helpful, supportive inner dialogue. We are talking not about suppressing thoughts and feelings but about acknowledging them and then changing them to more uplifting and outgoing thoughts. For success, you need to start *listening* to your thinking. When you become aware that you are thinking negatively, have an attitude of understanding and compassion toward yourself. Let go of those negative, restricting thoughts that include words such as *should, ought, must, always,* and *never;* they are limiting and always a put-down of either yourself or someone else. You can even say to yourself, "I have no need of these thoughts." Let the thoughts pass and then quickly move on to more positive thoughts. Any and every single moment in our lives is a turning point. We can either go along with a thought or change it, the choice is ours. We can choose to have thoughts that are supporting, realistic, and mood-enhancing.

## STOP AND CHANGE—HOW TO STOP NEGATIVE INNER TALK

There is a simple system to help you to change persistent negative thoughts, which is of *utmost importance* on your journey to natural pain relief. When you find discouraging, worrying thoughts in your mind and notice that you are listening to and agreeing with your negative inner voice, you can intervene in the following way.

*Say to yourself inside your head in a firm and convincing tone:*
"STOP!"

*You can use any other words that are really effective for you, such as* "STOP IT!" *or* "STOP THAT!" *Say or shout it really loud inside your head. You will find that there is an immediate stunned silence in your mind. You will have virtually shocked your thoughts into stopping for a moment or so. This negative voice isn't used to being ordered around; it generally has free rein! Now you can show it who is in charge. Don't give it a chance to get going again:* CHANGE *that old negative talk into a new supportive, positive voice. Immediately fill the silence with a more constructive thought.*

## Sample Affirmations for the Stop and Change Technique

*Select three or four of the following powerful and comforting positive sentences and have them ready to counter that negative voice. Choose statements that are meaningful to you and that resonate with you personally or, best of all, make up your own. Learn these positive replacement thoughts, or affirmations, as they are often called, by heart so they will always be ready for you.*

*"I am doing just fine."*

*"I am coping well."*

*"I love and approve of myself."*

*"I can handle this."*

*"It is easy for me to . . . (relax, be calm, cope, walk easily, sit comfortably, etc)."*

*"Be still, this will pass."* (a wonderful affirmation during a pain flare-up)

*"I am calm and confident."*

*"I am the power and authority in my life."*

*"I have the power and authority to release the past and accept my good now."*

*"I concentrate on what I can do."*

*"I am patient with myself and others."*

*"I respect my body."*

*"I am strong and my body is healing itself."*

*"I am filled with healing power."*

*"I deserve to be healthy."*

*"Today is a good day. Today is my day."*

If more negative thoughts come up when you first mentally say "STOP," tell them to stop again and replace them with your positive sentences once more. Don't let your good intentions be sabotaged; you now know better than to listen to that discouraging voice. Be persistent and keep replacing unhelpful negative thoughts with supporting thoughts until you are confident you have changed your inner voice to the positive again. Remember, *you* are in charge: your mind is only producing thoughts for you to deal with as you will, you don't *have* to listen to or be influenced by them. It is *your* choice. You can choose not to go along with negative thoughts, and instead to follow those thoughts you prefer. The real power is not with your thoughts because you can override them. The power is with *you*, with your wise inner self, the thinker behind the thoughts.

Write down your positive sentences for reference. Repeat your chosen phrases over and over until you feel yourself back in charge with a more positive outlook. Be prepared to change your affirmations as your needs and situation alter.

It is important to realize you don't have to *believe* the positive phrases initially. By saying your affirmations in a convincing tone of voice, either aloud or inside your head, you fool your subconscious mind into absorbing them. Your subconscious mind is not judgmental and always takes on board whatever messages it receives, whether the messages are true or false, negative or positive. This good news means you can feed your subconscious mind with all the most uplifting, constructive messages possible. They will be absorbed, the messages will be passed on, and your body and feelings will respond accordingly.

The Stop and Change technique is essential in gaining and retaining a positive attitude. It is easy, simple, and effective; the only part you have to work at is *remembering to do it*. With practice, you will gradually become more and more successful at noticing what you are thinking. In summary, an easy way to remember this technique is to remind yourself to—STOP AND CHANGE (STOP negative thoughts and CHANGE to positive thoughts).

## MORE ABOUT AFFIRMATIONS

Having a strong positive inner voice ready for action with meaningful affirmations is crucial to your success in the Stop and Change technique. You are aiming to train your mind to produce more positive thoughts automatically. You can look at the process of feeding affirmations into your subconscious mind as though your mind is a computer and you are the programmer. We feed our "mental computer" with information all the time and have done so all our life. Like other computers, we get back out only what we have put in. If we program our mental computer with positive thoughts, a more positive reality is bound to take place. The subconscious mind is also like a computer in the way that it doesn't care whether the information it is fed is true or false, which is why affirmations work so beautifully. Thus, we can choose to program our "computer mind" with thoughts supporting and uplifting us, giving us confidence, and making us feel better about ourselves—even if the affirmations are not true at the moment.

We are not deceiving ourselves by saying, for instance, "I am calm and confident," when it may be quite obvious that we are not. We are programming ourselves for what we want to achieve. For the very reason that our subconscious mind is so literal and accepts everything at face value, we *have* to say "I am calm and confident" as though we are calm and confident right now. This is because if we say "I want to be calm and confident" or "I will be calm and confident," our mind registers this as a future event, not a current situation, and so it will wait for the future to come. And we all know the future never comes. When we want to achieve a particular state, then, we have to word it in the present tense so our mind will accept it and start acting upon it.

Even if you are programming yourself with a particular future event in mind—for example, a doctor's appointment—you still need to have those feelings of confidence and calmness *now*. Your "computer mind" cannot tell the difference between imagined events and real ones. When you are thinking about a future event, your subconscious mind really does not know whether the meeting is taking place right now, at this very minute, or next week. So, if you are imagining the meeting taking place, as far as your subconscious mind is concerned, it is actually happening *now*. This is why you need to state your affirmations in the present tense. The word *affirm* means just this: that what we are saying is a fact, is already taking place. Set the scene by visualizing going through your appointment in a calm manner and say your affirmation at the same time, "I am calm and confident." Then, with constant repetition of the affirmation, when the time comes you will be set for success.

## Making Effective Affirmations

Affirmations can be about anything at all. You can work on any aspect of your life you like, from your health to your relationships (remembering you can change only *you;* you cannot change anyone else), your future hopes, the way you feel about yourself, giving up smoking, slimming, improving your confidence . . . just anything. For example, to help me in my program to improve my walking ability, I affirm "My back, hips, and legs are comfortable and strong, I walk freely and easily."

There are a few points to remember when making affirmations for yourself.

1. Make sure the outcome is one you really truly 100 percent desire.
2. Our minds are drawn toward what we think about and so always, always express affirmations in the *positive,* not the negative. For example, "I am calm and confident," *not* "I'm not worried." By using the first affirmation, your mind is drawn toward being calm and confident.
3. In order for your subconscious mind to accept them easily, keep affirmations *short* and *to the point.* Make it easy for your subconscious to accept them.
4. We are so used to complying with rules and regulations that sometimes it is easier to make affirmations in the form of an order—for example, "Stay calm" or "Walk freely and easily."
5. Repeat your affirmations over and over during the day, out loud if you can for maximum effect. By saying them aloud, the effect is more powerful. The more you can involve your whole body and its senses, the greater the impact will be. *Act* the affirmations as you say them for fastest and fullest effect. Involve your whole body and mind with the meaning of each affirmation. Think clearly about the meaning of the words and make a strong image in your mind of the affirmation actually being true of you.
6. Constant repetition is important. You need to impress your affirmations thoroughly upon your subconscious mind until the new thoughts begin to appear automatically.
7. Repeating affirmations can be particularly reassuring, uplifting, and mood-changing if used throughout times of stress or pain. You may

think, "How can I say 'I am calm and confident' when I'm not feeling like this right now?" Remember, it is not self-deception to make strong affirmations but rather *self-direction.* You are working to achieve the desired outcome.

8. You may see some results almost immediately; other changes may be more subtle and it may be some time before you notice changes taking place.

9. Sometimes it is surprisingly hard to repeat an affirmation. If you sense that one of your affirmations is meeting resistance, try this written exercise. *Take two pages, one for writing your affirmation and the opposite page for writing any response. As you write your affirmation, say it totally wholeheartedly to yourself. If any negative thoughts spring into your mind as you say the affirmation, write them down on the opposite page. Keep going until you have written your affirmation ten or more times. Look at the negative responses and create new affirmations to counter each one of them.*

The more you use your affirmations, the easier they become to accept and the more powerful an effect they have. Practice and practice as much as you can for a few weeks—and then you will find that you want to repeat the affirmations for the strength they bring you. Little by little, you will notice changes occurring in your life.

## Ideas for Using the Affirmations

- *Create a Power Pack by writing each sentence separately on small reminder cards, which are easy to handle. Keep the Power Pack of cards close to you, then you can memorize them at odd moments during the day.*
- *Read through your Power Pack early in the morning to set you up for the day. Say the affirmations out loud if possible, or inside your head.*
- *Read through the affirmations often during the day at quiet times, perhaps when you stop for some water or a cup of tea.*
- *Make a recording of affirmations to listen to as you work, drive, or walk. Say them, sing them, or chant them along with the tape, out loud if possible.*

- *Say your affirmations out loud while looking into a mirror. This is a very powerful technique. Say to your image, "You are calm and confident." Then say, "I am calm and confident." Notice how the two different statements make you feel. This method can double the impact of your affirmations.*
- *Read your Power Pack of affirmation cards through and then choose just one affirmation that seems particularly relevant at the moment. With this special affirmation you could:*

> *Write the affirmation on slips of paper and place them where you will see them often: around your workplace, car, or house; on mirrors, on the TV screen, on the fridge, for example.*
>
> *Keep writing this special affirmation over and over, as often as you like, repeating it to yourself at the same time.*
>
> *Draw a picture of the outcome of the affirmation. Make it big and bright and pin it up to remind you of your desired outcome.*

- *If you are having a particularly difficult day, read your affirmation cards every hour. You could set a timer to remind you if necessary. Or try making up new ones on, say, every hour (set your timer), write them down, and read them all through at the end of the day before you go to bed.*
- *Try reinforcing an affirmation in this way. "It is easy for me to . . . Yes, it is easy for me to . . ." (Insert your own particular need.)*

Never forget that what you believe about yourself can translate into reality. We are what we *believe* we are, so *refuse* to dwell on negative thoughts and *choose* to think supportive, constructive, and positive thoughts instead.

Choosing to concentrate on uplifting thoughts is one of the most important decisions you can make. Using affirmations, no matter what your current problems, will allow you to think well of yourself, to enjoy your life, to improve physical well-being, and, most of all, to cope with pain and feel in charge of your life.

## ACTION GUIDELINES

1. Try the two experiments Test Your Thoughts and Feelings, on page 21, and Test Your Muscles, on page 22.

2. Use the Stop and Change technique for handling your thoughts. Practice and more practice is the key to success.

3. Write supportive affirmations and make yourself a Power Pack on small reminder cards. Choose some ways of using them and use them every day.

# UNIT 3
∎
# Building Self-Esteem and a Positive Attitude

## CONTENTS

# Building Self-Esteem and a Positive Attitude

On those occasions when our confidence and self-esteem are high, we are happy with life as it is and content to be who we are. When we focus on the good things in life we feel balanced and calm. When we are full of joy and gratitude for what we have and, indeed, for life itself, we are fulfilled. In this harmonious state, everything we do appears simple and effortless: we are in touch with all our natural inner powers and strengths and life flows.

Whatever our situation, we can enjoy this balanced way of life more often. We can systematically build our confidence and sense of personal value. And, as our self-esteem grows, we benefit from increased vitality, joy, and free access to our inner wisdom. Increased positivity brings a more relaxed approach to life, which encourages reduced pain levels.

By developing a supporting, caring attitude to ourselves and our pain, the whole quality of our lives improves, enabling us to feel happier, more outgoing, and able to look to the future again. You, too, like many others caring for their pain, can enjoy a thriving and growing self-esteem and achieve balance in your life. As we learn to focus less on our pain, it can take its place in our lives at the side of the stage instead of in the spotlight.

From now on in our lives we are going to concentrate on developing an attitude of liking and approving of ourselves. We are going to use every opportunity to think well of ourselves and those around us. When we are in this positive frame of mind, we are in touch with our inner wisdom and strengths. This affects the whole quality and tone of our lives and allows us to see our pain in a different way. When we change our attitude toward the pain, it can result in the pain becoming tolerable, something we see as just part of our lives, something with which we can cope and something we can accommodate within our lives. Developing a positive attitude brings back hope, and enables us to affirm our future.

We can come to regard the part of our body that is giving us pain in another light. We can learn to:

Care for it instead of cursing it.
Try to help it instead of hating it.
Be more patient with it instead of getting angry about it.
Respect it instead of trying to force it to do what it cannot for the moment.

## BODY TALK

To assist us in this exciting journey of personal growth and discovery, we are going to find out more about how we "work." It is accepted that the thoughts we think have a direct influence on the way we feel and upon our body. This also happens in the reverse—*our body language can influence our thoughts.* In other words, the way in which we hold ourselves physically affects how we feel emotionally. You can see this for yourself in this quick experiment.

- *Take a moment to notice how you are feeling right now. What are your emotions? Whatever they are, just make a mental note of them.*
- *Now let your shoulders sag forward, the corners of your mouth go down, your chin drop, and your head droop down.*
- *Notice how you are feeling now. Can you feel the difference?*

Quickly go on to the next experiment to dispel any negative sensations.

- *This time, relax your eyes, put a smile on your face, raise your arms (taking care to move only as far as is comfortable), and face as though toward the sun.*

- *Notice how you feel now.*
- *Did you feel the difference between the two body postures?*

In doing this experiment we were only "acting" but, although we may not have felt in a particularly negative or positive mood, our emotions were affected by the pose we took. When our body language said "I feel uplifted," we actually experienced a fleeting sensation of being uplifted emotionally.

Actors themselves demonstrate another example of this effect as they often "take their work home." Acting a part can affect them personally, influencing their own behavior. Some actors in long-running parts have acknowledged that their personality has been altered considerably by the part they are playing. If they are acting the part of a miserable, depressed person, they themselves may become more inward-looking than they may otherwise have been. Conversely, when acting the part of a happy-go-lucky type, actors may become more lighthearted themselves.

This information is exciting for us, as we can use it in our own cause. By using positive body language and acting in a positive manner, we can influence our mind into responding accordingly. Thus, by acting "my life is joyful," the feelings will follow; we will become and feel more joyful. The next exercise, based on the ideas above, is most liberating and empowering, enabling us to become more confident and relaxed, thereby reducing our discomfort.

### *"How Would it Be if I Was . . . ?"*

*Take five minutes or so to sit or lie down quietly where you won't be disturbed. Become aware of your breathing and notice the gentle rise and fall of your body as you breathe in and out. On your next out breath, let your breath out through your mouth with a slight sigh.*

*On the next out breath, imagine the sigh going down from the top of your head to the soles of your feet. As you let all the air go, feel the tension drain away.*

*Now that you're relaxed, continue to breathe normally. Take your attention around your body, relaxing each part as you become aware of it: your feet, your legs, your abdomen, your lower back, then up your back to your shoulders and neck, and then all around your face and head.*

*And now bring to mind a situation where you feel you need support or help in some way, a situation about which you may have negative feelings. Ask yourself,* "How would it be if I was a confident, optimistic person?"

*Imagine yourself acting as if you were confident and optimistic and see how you would behave in that situation. Ask yourself lots of questions, such as:*

"*How would I look?*"
"*What would I be feeling?*"
"*How would I be moving?*"
"*How would I be dressed?*"
"*Where would I be?*"
"*Would anyone be with me?*"
"*How would other people react to me?*"
"*What would I do?*"
"*What would I do next?*"
"*What would the outcome be?*"

*Keep saying to yourself* "If I was confident and optimistic I would . . ." *as you imagine taking part in the situation upon which you are working.*

*Watch yourself in the situation, feeling good, handling everything as though you were a confident and optimistic person.*

*Enjoy these powerful feelings for a while before you come back to the room. When you are ready to get up, stretch yourself and take the feelings you have created with you. Know that you can have these feelings in any situation at any time if you act as though you were that confident person.*

*You can use this exercise for other qualities also. For example, you could say,* "How would it be if I was a calm person?" *or* "How would it be if I was good at controlling my pain?"

*Choose words that feel right for you and are relevant to each particular situation you want to work upon.*

As we go through this imaginative exercise, we find that by acting "confidence," we become confident. Of course, we have achieved this in our imagination, but now that we have experienced the feeling inside, we have given ourselves the power to be able to carry the actions through in real life in any situation we choose. Keep practicing this exercise, and when you are in a real-life situation, recall how you felt during the imaginative work. You will have the power to bring your visualized actions to life.

Once you are experienced with the technique, you can use it spontaneously, at any time you find yourself feeling uncertain or in a negative frame of mind. Just ask yourself, "How would it be if I was a . . . [insert desired quality here] . . . person?" Your wise inner self knows the answer, and by asking, you release the inner power to act in that way. This is an important and transforming exercise and can have a great impact on your whole way of being.

## KEEP SMILING

When you acted the body movements of "joy" in the experiment at the beginning of this unit (see pages 37–38), the biggest factor in the uplifting of your feelings was the smile you put on your face. Smiling uses fewer muscles than do unhappy expressions, and when you smile your face widens and relaxes. The muscles of our face regulate the flow of blood to our brain. Smiling allows blood to flow freely to our brain, where all the cells receive an increased supply of nutrients, enabling them to function efficiently. It is now known that laughing and smiling activate the production of endorphins, our bodies' natural painkillers. When smiling, we use fewer muscles and benefit from the extra oxygen we are receiving, our brainpower is improved, and we look and feel younger. By deliberately putting a smile on your face, you can immediately boost your mood. You don't have to *feel* like smiling; the smile itself sends positive messages to your subconscious mind, which automatically passes them on to your body. Remember as you get dressed in the morning—the first thing you don is a smile.

## The Inner Smile

To continue with this theme, try the lovely Inner Smile visualization. Make sure you will be undisturbed for anything between five and twenty minutes for this relaxation. Take off your shoes and loosen any tight clothing. Sit or lie down in a position that is as comfortable as possible for you. When you go through the relaxation, do allow plenty of time with each part of your body.

1. *Become aware of your breathing and just notice the gentle rise and fall of your body as you breathe in and out. On your next out breath, let your breath out through your mouth with a slight sigh. Let there be just a hint of a smile about your face; the smile will help to relax your whole face. Breathe in through your nose.*

   *On the next out breath, imagine the sigh going down from the top of your head to the soles of your feet. As you let the air go, feel the tension drain away.*

   *Continue to breathe normally.*

2. *Now you are going to take your attention to different parts of your body in turn, starting with your abdomen. As you breathe in, imagine your breath going down to that area and filling it with warmth and healing energy. Feel your abdomen being bathed in nourishing oxygen and sense that all the cells in that area are refreshed and working well. Know they are happy with the attention you are giving them. Imagine all the tiny cells laughing and jiggling about. And then sense the whole of the area smiling. Imagine a smile from one side of your abdomen to the other. As you imagine your abdomen smiling, it will respond by widening and relaxing even more. Stay with this image for as long as you want to.*

3. *Repeat Step 2 for as many other parts of your body as you have time. Areas that will particularly benefit from this attention are your back, your neck, and your face, of course. You may also feel able to approach the part that hurts in this way; it will encourage your natural healing processes.*

4. *When you have completed your relaxation, lie still for a while in the wonderful warm, relaxed, and happy glow you will have created and know that this sensation is there, waiting for you, at any time.*

5. *When you are ready to get up, stretch yourself and take the feelings you have created with you, keeping a gentle smile on your face, knowing your whole body is smiling on the inside.*

## THE TREASURE STORE

Gathering together a Treasure Store of self-esteem is of absolute top priority on your journey to natural pain relief. With the Treasure Store exercise, you are going to amass your own personal nest egg of "gold." You will need a personal notebook to collect your "treasure." The notebook can take any form: an ordinary exercise book, an attractive journal, a diary, or a file. Whatever you select, make it a book just for you and your personal notes. It is going to be your own treasure trove of positivity to support you on your way. The Treasure Store will become a collection of ideas, techniques that you find effective, and your own achievements and successes. You can use it to record your work on the techniques in this book. In times of need, you will be able to raid your treasure for inspiration and support.

The Treasure Store notebook is an ongoing project, and it can be used for recording and working on any of the following areas, plus anything else you choose—it is *your* treasure.

- Jotting down techniques you find helpful
- Working your way through techniques
- Noting ways in which you cope with the pain
- Entering achievements and successes
- Exploring and releasing your feelings
- Writing down your thoughts
- Recording and working through your daily concerns
- Writing affirmations
- Recording your body exercise program
- Expressing hopes and wishes for the future
- Recording visualizations
- Noting goals and your progress toward them
- Exploring significant events

- Recording and interpreting dreams
- Expressing yourself through drawings

Get into the habit of using your Treasure Store notebook every day, whether for reading about your progress, for refreshing your memory about uplifting ideas and techniques, or for writing a new entry. Keep the book near you and let it become a source of nourishment. The increase in your sense of self-worth will be boundless when you have such a stash of treasure behind you. You will gain understanding and insight into your pain. It will, most important of all, help you to gain a sense of control in your life. Your image of yourself will expand and your self-value increase abundantly.

## GO FOR GOLD

The one vital ingredient in developing a positive attitude is to build your self-confidence. Self-confidence comes from having respect for yourself, seeing value in yourself, accepting yourself just as you are (warts and all), and liking and approving of yourself.

Go for Gold, an exercise for fostering awareness of positive attitudes, is your first entry in your storehouse of positivity. When we actively seek positive attitudes in our world, we find that they rub off on to us without any effort. On your journey to increased confidence, make a deliberate plan to seek out the good in all you see. You sometimes may have to seek very diligently at first until you become accustomed to the idea of homing in on the good things of life, but it will soon become easier and easier. For instance, it's rarely helpful to search the news on the radio or television each day for an attitude of joy. Aim always for constructive, uplifting input into your life and choose to surround yourself with that which is good. Start now with building your own treasure trove of inner strength. Your "gold" is all the tiny nuggets of good you can find anywhere around or within you. When you collect all of these together, they will accumulate until you have a treasure trove of positivity overflowing around you.

*For your first valuable "deposit" in your Treasure Store, write down all the positive attitudes and occurrences that come to your attention in your daily life. It does not matter how small the incident. These could be things people say and do, phrases from books, the names of inspiring pieces of music—in fact, anything that you find lifts and supports you. It is a good idea to do this every day if possible, as you would in keeping a diary. Keep on adding to your lists as you notice life-enhancing events around you, wherever you happen to be.*

*Make two lists, side by side. On one side note the incident and on the other side write the positive attribute. An example is:*

| The Incident | The Positive Attitude I Feel |
|---|---|
| A friend came to see me | friendly |
| | happy |
| Sang in my shower | exhilarated |
| Watched comedy show on TV | amused |
| | relaxed |
| Listened to the birds in the garden | peaceful |
| | joyful |
| | healthy |
| Did my exercises | pleased with myself |
| | invigorated |
| Read book | inspired |
| Made a long-awaited decision | content |

Keep your notebook near you so you can continue to add to your treasure, and reread it often. If you are feeling discouraged and need a special lift, boost your mood by reading the list of positive attitudes you have felt. Read the list aloud if you like and before each word start with "I am . . ." For example, say "I am grateful," "I am helpful," . . . and so on down the list.

Say each sentence wholeheartedly, even if you don't feel that particular emotion to begin with. By the time you have completed the list, you will feel yourself uplifted. Your subconscious mind does not differentiate between "real" thoughts and the thoughts you deliberately place in your mind. It does not matter if the thoughts are true or not; the subconscious mind just acts on the information fed to it. What an advantage for us! So speak with conviction, and your mind will take the messages on board and your body will respond accordingly.

## "WHAT A STAR!"

We all thrive and grow in confidence in an atmosphere of approval and praise. Who better for it to come from than the person who knows us best—ourself? We sometimes forget that it is not only children who need and deserve praise in order to grow in confidence and self-esteem: adults deserve it too. Yes, *deserve* praise. *You* deserve praise, you are worthy of praise. You may feel you haven't done anything special, but you don't *need* to do anything special. You are special already. You and I each have unique abilities, skills, and qualities. Mine are different from yours and yours are different from everyone else's in the world. As we learn to value the tiniest aspect of our personality and ability, our confidence will grow and flourish.

You will need your new personal notebook, your Treasure Store, for this exercise for burnishing your self-image and praising and valuing yourself. When you gain in personal confidence, you will find that others respond to you in a positive way and you will bloom and blossom in this supporting, uplifting atmosphere.

*In your notebook, make a long list of all the qualities you like about yourself (at least twenty), including skills you have learned and physical characteristics. Head the page with "What a Star!" if you like; it will make you smile and remind you what the exercise is all about—making you feel good. To start you off, review your Go for Gold lists for ideas.*

*To make the list of even more value to you, write a sentence about each quality with an idea of how you use that particular attribute. For example:*

## WHAT A STAR!

| My Qualities | How I Use My Qualities |
|---|---|
| *I am a good cook* | *I enjoy cooking special dinners* |
| *I am a good organizer* | *I plan all our finances* |
| *I've been told I have a lovely smile* | *I will use my smile more often!* |
| *I am enthusiastic about helping the environment* | *I recycle all my cans and paper* |
| *I am determined* | *My determination will help me keep to my new pain plan* |

*Read your list through often and add to it when you can.*

The list can be used in different ways:

- You can read across, linking the two sides with "and."
- Read just one side or the other.
- Expand the list by thinking of different uses for each of your qualities. The list will then be updated and relevant each time you read it, for instance:

  On the first reading:
  *"I am a good organizer and I plan all our finances."*
  On the second reading:
  *"I am a good organizer and I am taking care of our menus and shopping lists."*
  On the third reading:
  *"I am a good organizer and I am planning lists of plants for the new bed in the garden."*
  . . . and so on.

By working regularly with the two exercises Go for Gold and "What a Star!" in your personal notebook, you will find that your confidence grows and grows. Seek every chance to cultivate an atmosphere of positivity around you and within you. Your growing self-esteem will set you up for coping with your pain in a new, dynamic way.

# THE CULTIVATION OF APPRECIATION

Another wonderfully simple factor in entering a balanced and happy state is the cultivation of an attitude of appreciation in our lives. Whatever our condition, there are always many positive aspects in our lives for us to value. Often, in our concern over our physical state, we may have neglected to see all the good around us. However, when we focus on and become more sensitive to all the good things in our lives and all the things we *can* do, we will find we experience more joy in our lives. Positive thoughts draw more positive thoughts to them, happiness attracts more happiness, and so our bounty will grow and grow.

Transform your attitude toward your pain and your situation by regularly using the following exercises.

## *The Golden Bubble*

The first exercise is to search out those tiny nuggets of gold in your daily life in a bedtime review. Spend a few minutes last thing at night preparing for a peaceful night's sleep with a visual diary by thinking back through your day, searching out every tiny nugget to add to your hoard of treasure. This exercise will further enhance your positive attitude, as it has an expansive ending, where you reach out to others, sharing your treasure with them.

*Take a few minutes for the Golden Bubble before you go to sleep. Start by paying attention to your breathing, just noticing the rise and fall of your body. Allow your breathing to become slightly slower and deeper. After a few moments, on your next out breath, allow your breath to float out with a slight sigh. Feel all the tension drain out of you down into the surface beneath you. On your next out breath, allow the sigh to go from the top of your head to the bottom of your feet.*

*And now that you are relaxed, think back, gently gathering all the tiny snippets of "good" from your day, all the blessings and magical moments. It may be someone's smile, a letter, compliments you have received or given, a beautiful sky, an enjoyable program, a phone call, a visit, a touch, the smell and color of some fruit, the way you handled your pain at a certain time, a "thank-you," your meal—absolutely everything that enhanced your day and made your heart expand. Linger over each little item, savor it, and bring it back to your mind in great detail, with any of the associated senses, such as colors, sounds, tastes, textures, smells.*

*When you have amassed all your gold, you will find that there is a sensation of warmth, joy, and gratitude within you.*

*Now you are going to give this wonderful gift to someone else who may benefit from this comfort. This gift has magical qualities; when we give away those feelings of warmth and love, they do not all depart, with none left for ourselves; we actually retain a growing abundance of warmth and love inside our own hearts and minds. In giving, our own feelings of love and gratitude grow.*

*Imagine this feeling of warmth and goodwill is transformed into a wonderful golden light. See in your mind's eye the golden light enclosed inside a beautiful golden bubble. Now send the bubble containing the golden light to spread warmth and golden light to someone else who would benefit from this comfort. See the bubble sparkling and glowing as it floats away up into the sky. Watch it become smaller and smaller. Say a big thank-you of gratitude to all those golden moments of your day as you watch it float off. Now imagine it arriving at its destination and watch as the bubble dissolves, surrounding the person to whom you have sent it with golden light, warmth, and love.*

*This imaginative exercise will set you up for a wonderful, peaceful night with sweet dreams and a sense of thankfulness and appreciation for your life.*

This creative exercise is especially important for people like us who may feel we are no longer able to contribute to others as much as we did in the past.

## Waking Up

You may want to try this and the following exercise, which are excellent additions to the previous exercises. Waking Up continues with the same theme as The Golden Bubble and is aimed at programming you and setting the atmosphere for the coming day.

> *Make your very first thoughts each day positive and appreciative. Make a new habit of praising and valuing your life and everything in it each morning as you awake.*
>
> *As soon as you wake, make a mental list of at least six of the good things in your life. You can include anything from your lovely warm bed to all the things you can do. You will find your heart expands as gratitude floods in. The sensation of warmth and expansion will flow into your day, giving you a wonderful start.*

## Thank You

The words *thank you* are an expression of gratitude and appreciation. A wonderful way to maintain the morning glow from your Waking Up exercise is to do the Thank You exercise as often as you want during the day. I find this exercise especially helpful at stressful times. It is good to acknowledge our good fortune in the many other areas of our lives.

> *You can do this exercise while you are lying down, sitting, or moving around. You could choose from any of the following phrases or express your thanks in your own way. The words you use don't matter as much as the desire to show that you value the small things of life.*
>
> *"Thank you . . ." [the name of the object] or "I am grateful for . . ."*
> *or "Thanks be for . . ."*
> *or "Thank you for . . ."*
> *or "I am fortunate that . . ."*
> *or "I appreciate . . ."*
>
> *Examples when looking out or being outside:*
>
> *"I appreciate the sky."*

*"I appreciate the trees."*
*"I appreciate the grass."*
*"I appreciate these flowers."*
*"I appreciate being able to sense all these things."*

*Carry on adding to your mental list until you are filled with the blessings of life.*

When we do this exercise wholeheartedly, we find that by concentrating on and valuing what we *have,* we are filled with a sensation of love and warmth with appreciation for life itself.

Now, this may sound like a simplistic exercise, but it is, in fact, very powerful—so do try it. Remember—it is worth trying *anything* we can to keep our minds aimed toward positivity.

## A POSITIVE ATTITUDE TO YOUR PAIN

Within us there is a powerful healing force striving continually to repair our body. This force operates most efficiently when we are relaxed and feeling good. Knowing this, we can appreciate that in addition to developing our self-esteem and general confidence, we best support ourselves by developing a positive, caring attitude toward our pain. We do this by trying to help our body in whatever ways we can, being patient with ourselves and the hurting part, and respecting our body for what it can and cannot do at the moment. We can learn to get in contact with our pain, not cursing or fighting it but caring for it, befriending it. We can speak with compassion and understanding directly to the part of our body concerned and thank it for everything it has done in the past. We can tell the area that we understand it is hurt at the moment, and we are doing the best we can to help it.

*For example, a positive conversation with a hurt back could go something like this:*

*"Thank you for everything you have done for me in the past. I'm so sorry if I have mistreated you. I know you are hurting now and I'm doing my best to help you and*

*care for you. Please let me know if there is anything you need: I am listening."*

*If you take all your attention into the hurt area and speak to it in your own way, you may very well receive a message. It could be a feeling, a thought, or a picture that comes to your mind. Be open and take notice of the very first sensations that come to you; this is how your wise inner self communicates with you. If there is no feedback from your body at this time, just spend a few minutes breathing warmth and relaxation into the part that hurts; this will also let the area know you are caring for it. Try to contact the part again on another occasion very soon. Continue to use this technique to foster a caring relationship with your body.*

As the relationship grows, our respect for our body increases and we are less likely to mistreat it. In caring for our body in this positive way, we gain further opportunities for pain-reducing endorphins to flow and for healing to take place.

The more we use the techniques in this book, the more our confidence will grow. The more our confidence increases, the more we feel in charge of our pain and are able to look to the future again. The pain will begin to take its place in our lives at the side of the stage instead of in the limelight.

## ACTION GUIDELINES

1. Work on boosting your confidence every day. Use the ideas from this unit to help you. Success depends upon both the way you approach your pain and the techniques you use. Try these exercises wholeheartedly—and they will work. A positive attitude will keep you on course with all your self-help work—an attitude of "I don't know if it will work, but I'll give it my best effort."

2. Most important: start your own personal journal, your Treasure Store of positivity. Get into the habit of keeping your Treasure Store of inspiration close to you. You will gain support and confidence from your own descriptions of your self-worth.

3. Give yourself plenty to look forward to. (See Unit 8, Enjoying Yourself, for exercises that will help you with this.)

4. See Unit 2, What Are You Telling Yourself? for information about stopping negative thoughts and replacing them with positive ones.

5. *Remember always to concentrate your mind on what you* CAN *do and change your attitude to one of appreciation of what you do have.*

# UNIT 4
■
# Pictures in Your Mind

## CONTENTS

# Pictures in Your Mind

We can make an almost magical transformation to our life, and to the healthy functioning of our body, by the conscious and creative use of our imagination. When we use our imagination with flair and skill, we can achieve wonders. This is one of the most exciting and powerful techniques available to us.

Anyone and everyone has the ability to use his or her imagination in a creative way, although it is a skill that may have been forgotten. When we were children, we would normally spend hours using our imagination in a fantasy world, playacting or daydreaming. As we grew up, we may have been told to stop daydreaming and encouraged instead to use our powers of reasoning. This was often at the expense of our creativity, the source of which is in the right side of our brain, our powers of logic lying on the left side. When we are perfectly in balance, we use both sides of our brain equally, combining left-brain logic and right-brain imagination. As an adult, we may not have used this natural power for many, many years, but with practice the ability can soon be revived and nurtured.

When we use our imagination for a positive input into our life, it is often known as creative visualization, positive visualization, or creative imagery. A study of visualization has been done in America. Three groups of people had their performance measured when goal-shooting at a basketball net. One group practiced for twenty minutes a day, another group did not practice at all, and the third group *imagined* practicing their goal-shooting skills. After twenty days, each group's performance was tested again. As expected, the group that did not practice had not improved at all. The group that had practiced their skills improved by 24 percent. The big news was that those who did nothing but visualize shooting goals had improved by 23 percent, virtually the same as those who had practiced in reality. Similar results were found in experiments with other sporting activities.

This particular research was with sporting skills, but the same findings apply to many other aspects of our life. This exciting discovery proved what many people knew already: our mind is powerful and can affect the way our body functions. We do not physically have to be somewhere or physically do something for our subconscious mind to believe that the event is actually taking place. When we deliberately use visualization to change some aspect of our life, we are feeding messages to our subconscious mind. The subconscious mind accepts what it is sent, whether the messages come from our thoughts, from affirmations, or from visualized, imagined pictures. This part of our mind does not have a logical aspect to it, nor does it question the information it receives. For example, the subconscious minds of the goal shooters did not know whether the men were shooting goals in reality or not; they just registered the accurate shooting of the goals. The men who did not practice goal-shooting but trained with their minds only used visualization skills. After relaxing, they concentrated their minds, pictured the whole action in detail, and told themselves they could successfully score goals. This visualization convinced their subconscious minds that the goal-shooting was actually happening at that moment. As a result, their minds sent the appropriate information to their bodies, giving a positive outcome.

If we see clearly in our minds what we want, the reality will follow; it is as simple as that. When we use our imaginative skills, the pictures we "see" are immediately translated into physical or emotional reality with a speed as instant as switching on a light. This has wonderful meaning for us. We can harness this power to our own good to make the changes we desire and thus have a real input into bringing healing to ourselves and reducing our pain.

## PRACTICING VISUALIZATION SKILLS

We already use the skill of visualization in our daily lives even though we may not recognize it as such. Whenever we do anything, we first of all see the event in our mind as a picture, although the process may be so fast that we are unaware that it takes place. For instance, if you have ever planned a holiday, browsing through brochures and thinking of how you will enjoy the time, you will have seen, albeit fleetingly, pictures in your mind first.

### Step 1

Try recalling the events listed below and notice if you see a picture in your mind or receive some other sensation in your body. There is absolutely no need to *try* to do or see anything. If you receive images or sensations, that's fine; if you don't, that's okay too. We cannot *force* images and sensations upon ourselves. Allow yourself to relax, take your time with each suggestion, and just notice what happens.

Recall:

> *The sound of a car passing by*
> *The sensation of rain falling on your hand*
> *The sound of chalk on a blackboard*
> *The texture of toast in your mouth*
> *The smell of coffee*
> *The sensation of running*
> *Stroking a cat*
> *A rainbow*
> *Reaching up to pick blackberries*
> *A blue sky and a turquoise sea*
> *The smell of an orange*

You will probably have seen, heard, or sensed the response in some way, however fleetingly.

### Step 2

The next stage is to practice your imaginative skills with each of your senses individually.

*Imagine objects you know really well; include all the senses, those of sight, hearing, touch, taste, and smell and that of movement. Take your time with each suggestion and just allow sensations to come. Once again, relax and don't try to receive anything.*

**Sight.** *See a picture of a yellow banana, a pink rose, a green baseball field, a blue sky with white clouds, a setting sun, a red traffic light.*

**Hearing.** *Hear the sound of birds singing, an airplane overhead, a bell, water running into a bath, a kettle boiling, the telephone ringing, a newspaper rustling.*

**Touch.** *Feel the sensation of stroking an animal, touching a thistle, your hand in a stream of water, touching the top of a wooden gate, a rubber ball in your hand, holding a metal bar.*

**Taste.** *Taste in your mouth a lemon, soft ice cream, a favorite drink, salt and vinegar chips, a juicy apple.*

**Smell.** *Smell the aroma of freshly baked bread, coffee, a rose, a ripe melon, a bonfire.*

**Movement.** *Feel the sensation in your body of hopping, riding a bike, swimming, chopping vegetables, skipping, running, picking up a heavy weight.*

## Step 3

To develop your visualization skills further, make up a short scene for yourself using as many of your senses as you can. It would be a good idea to use the images you have already practiced in the previous exercise and combine some of them together in the story. This will help you to receive as full and clear a picture as possible. Here is an example of a simple visualization using some of the practiced images. If you choose to use this short visualization, you may want to record it yourself or ask someone to read it to you.

*Make yourself comfortable, allow your breathing to become quiet and a little slower and deeper. Feel any tension drain out of you. Let go of expectations and be prepared to accept whatever happens. See yourself in the scene, as though everything is happening to you. Make the scene as big, bright, colorful, and full of sounds as you can, using all your senses. Take your time with each part of the story.*

*Imagine that you are getting up in the morning. . . . You turn on the shower, hear the sound of the water flowing. . . . You put your hand in to test the temperature and then have your shower, feeling the contact of the water as it cascades over you. . . . Later, you fill a kettle and listen for the sound of it boiling . . . and you make a hot drink. . . . You smell and taste it. . . . You leave home to catch a bus. As you walk along the path, you smell the acrid smoke from a neighbor's bonfire. Overhead you notice an airplane with a vapor trail slowly making its way over the beautiful blue sky. . . . You flag down your bus . . . and jump on to it. . . . You feel the sensation of the cold, hard metal handrail under your hands . . . and hear the rustle of the passengers' newspapers. As the bus pulls off, you feel the jerky movement reflected in your body. . . . When you reach your destination, you jump down from the bus . . . and are greeted by the smell of newly baked bread from a nearby bread shop. . . . You are tempted by the smell and go inside and see and smell the display of pastries, buns, rolls, loaves, and cakes. . . . You buy yourself a favorite treat and savor every mouthful as you go along your way. . . . You feel happy and relaxed. And now, as you quietly come back to the room, bring the sensations of happiness and relaxation with you. Keep them with you as you continue with your day.*

You may find some of the sensations to be clearer than others. This is perfectly normal, as we all have one or two senses that are stronger than the others. Some people may see images vividly and others are able to hear sounds clearly. Don't necessarily expect to see long-lasting pictures in your mind, as though on a TV screen. The scene may come to you in a flash or just as *knowing* you are running, *knowing* you are touching a metal handrail.

## *Step 4*

The previous visualization comes mostly from our current memories of objects and events we have seen and sensations we have felt. The next stage in developing our visualization skills is to move on to more creative, imaginary scenes. Try this out in a very simple way at first. The technique is good fun, which is always a bonus for us, so just relax: don't think about *how* you are doing or whether you are being successful. In fact, don't concern yourself with the outcome at all. The essence of successful visualization is to be open and receptive and to let whatever will come, come, without concerning yourself about whether it is "right" or "good enough."

When we use our visualization skills to create these relaxing scenes in our mind, they are most effective when we relax our body and mind first with a short relaxation session. This gives the imaginative side of our brain freedom to roam and be inventive: freedom from the questioning, logical side of our brain. Once again, you may prefer to either record the script or have someone read it to you. Visualization skills are also practiced on the CD that accompanies this book. Even if you choose to listen to the CD, it will still be helpful to read through the exercise below.

*Be where you can be comfortable, free from distraction and disturbance, and allow your breathing to become quiet and slow. . . . On your next out breath, allow your body to relax. . . . On your next out breath, allow your mind to relax, letting go of any thoughts as they come to your notice; they need not concern you now. . . . This is your time—your time to be peaceful and to enjoy yourself. Let pictures or sensations come to you without forcing or trying. If they don't come, keep on relaxing and concentrate on your breath for a while and just see what happens. . . .*

*Imagine that you are lying at the base of a beautiful tree on the green grass. Feel the ground beneath you, warm and firm. You hear birds singing above you in the tree. A gentle summer breeze ruffles the leaves of the tree slightly . . . and you feel the sensation of the breeze lightly on your skin. . . . The light is dappled and you feel relaxed and content. Look up at the blue sky: there are no clouds, and it is a perfect day. And now imagine that your name appears, one letter at a time, in big letters in the sky. Each letter is a different color when it appears. Just watch each letter appear and allow the colors to come spontaneously. When each letter appears, hear a bright tinging sound, as though a magic wand has tapped the letter into being. When your whole name is in the sky, imagine hearing a fanfare being played. It is being played to announce, recognize, and honor you. Feel proud to be who you are, feel at one with the world, and know you are an important part of the whole universe. Slowly become aware of the surface beneath you and gently bring yourself back to the room, retaining those wonderful feelings as you quietly start movement again.*

## Step 5

When we were children, we let our imaginations run free, creating all kinds of fantasies and adventures. We often playacted at "being" various people and things. Involve yourself in the following experiences and rediscover the joys of an uninhibited imagination.

Take your time over these role-play activities. There's no need to try them all at once; spread them out over a few days if you want. You may experience these visualizations sitting or lying down to relax, or, if you like, move your body as well and really *be* the parts as you play them.

*Visualize wholeheartedly the objects, animals, and people on the list below and let your imagination run wild. Play these roles in your mind totally and completely, sensing everything about being that particular person, animal, or thing. You aren't looking at, say, a fish; you are that fish. Make the most of each one; see and feel what you would look like, whether you have clothes or fur, and so on, hear what is happening, what things feel like. For example, if you are the washing on a line, what do the clothespins feel like? What do the sun and wind feel like? If you are a mouse, what do your whiskers feel like? What is it like to have a tail? What are you eating, seeing, hearing, and doing, and how do you move?*

*Have fun and BE . . .*

*a fish*
*a growing seed*
*a goblin*
*a washing machine*
*an airplane*
*some washing on a line on a windy day*
*a mouse*
*an eagle*
*a newspaper*
*a king or a queen*

## Developing Your Skills

Practice all your new visualization skills during the day and last thing at night before you go to sleep. It is a good idea to continue with all these visualization exercises, and to make up some of your own for further practice. Experiment with bringing faces and scenes to life. Visualize to music. Visualize being different people—be creative. Put yourself in situations you would normally never find yourself—playing in the World Cup final, paddling up the Amazon, hang gliding—or find yourself in a completely innovative world of fantasy. Bring all your senses into play to foster development of your creative, imaginative mind.

The most effective visualizations, especially when you come to using the process for helping your body, are those you create for yourself to suit your personality and your own needs. Now that you've developed some visualization skills, you can move on to create your own visualization, a visualization that will be the foundation for many others and which you can use on many different occasions. This personal visualization can be used as a starting point when you need to relax, when you want to withdraw to think about a problem, to encourage peaceful sleep, to "rehearse" forthcoming events, to gain success with your goals, to give you confidence or other positive feelings, or when you want to create a fantasy adventure.

## SAFE HAVEN VISUALIZATION

You are going to create your own personal visualization in your mind, a place for yourself where you can feel safe and relaxed. This place is very special and just for you, somewhere you can feel peaceful and happy. It could be somewhere you know, some favorite spot, or it could be an imaginary place, perhaps a beautiful enclosed garden, a beach, a woodland glade, a hill overlooking the surrounding countryside, a penthouse apartment overlooking a city, a little country cottage, a riverboat, or it could be somewhere that is a complete fantasy, such as an underwater cave or on a star. Make it your very own space for you and you alone. No one else can enter this private world unless you choose to invite him in. Use all your senses and make your haven very clear in your mind; imagine the decoration, the surroundings, the sounds you may hear, and all the associated sensations. Take your time and spend anything from five to twenty minutes on enjoying the visualization. Here is an example of how you could go about it. A variation of the Safe Haven Visualization, called The Sanctuary, is also on the CD accompanying this book. If you choose to listen to the CD, it will still be helpful to read through the exercise below. Alternatively, you may record the script yourself or have it read slowly to you, leaving plenty of pauses, especially where you see the dots.

> *Make sure you are comfortable, warm, and in a quiet space of your own. Take your attention to your breath and allow it to become slightly slower and deeper. . . . Feel your body become relaxed, still, and quiet. . . . Allow the relaxation to spread throughout your body. . . . When thoughts come into your mind, let them go without following them. . . . Spend a few minutes relaxing in this way, enjoying the sensations and peace you have created . . . and then begin your visualization.*
>
> *Imagine you are on a little path leading to a beautiful place of your very own that brings immediate feelings of calmness and serenity. . . . Have a strong sense of your surroundings. Is it indoors or outdoors? . . . This is a special place. . . . Look around where you are and enjoy every detail of your safe haven. . . .*

*Notice the colors around you. . . . the sounds . . . what you feel
beneath you and around you. . . . What are you wearing? . . .
What are you doing? . . . Feel relaxed, peaceful, and happy to
be where you are. . . . Have somewhere you can sit or lie down
comfortably . . . and somewhere to keep writing materials . . .
paints or anything else you may want to use from time to time
to express your feelings. . . .*

*Feel yourself restored, with peace of mind. . . . Now explore
your surroundings and see yourself moving freely and strongly
. . . with a spring and bounce in your walk . . . enjoying
sparkling good health . . . doing all you would like to do . . .
achieving your goals and dreams, easily and successfully. . . .
You feel confident . . . vibrant . . . and fully alive. . . happy to be
who you are.*

*Continue to explore the nooks and crannies of your special
space and enjoy your positive feelings until it is time for you to
return along the same path as you came, and then, gently and
slowly, come back to the room. Bring back the feelings with you
to support you throughout the day, or, if it is bedtime, continue
to relax and daydream and let yourself drift off into a full night
of peaceful sleep.*

Visit your haven often and bring more detail to it each time you visit.
You will find your Safe Haven Visualization so precious that you will
want to use it on many occasions. You will be able to escape to it when
you need comfort or uplifting or increased confidence and for the natural pain relief that is often the outcome. You will be able to use it as the
basis for many future visualizations.

You may have noticed there is a strong emotional content in this
visualization. Feelings of peace and tranquillity are evoked, along with
strong feelings of being healthy, happy, and confident. When we bring
our emotions into the visualization, it is strengthened, and clear, strong
messages are sent to our subconscious mind. Remember the basketball
players? They added to their goal-shooting visualization the will to
succeed and felt the sensations of success within themselves that later
translated into the reality of success. The input of our positive emotions

to the visualization ensures a successful outcome. We are not deceiving ourselves with these imagined successes and sensations; we are directing and determining the outcome.

## VISUALIZATIONS FOR PAIN RELIEF

You may be aware I have not referred to pain during any of these visualizations. You probably have found that pain levels drop because you have relaxed your body and sent your mind on imaginative journeys and explorations, both of which help the healing process. This is a splendid discovery, and you may find that the pain relief you obtain is perfectly adequate. However, you can have an even more direct input into pain reduction with the help of certain images and some variations upon the basic technique.

### Pain Relief with Images of Water

Many people discover that, for them, images of their pain flowing out of them like water are the most effective. You can easily incorporate water images into your basic Safe Haven Visualization. For example, once you have relaxed and entered your special place and spent some time there enjoying it, you could continue the visualization and imagine any of the following scenes:

> *Stand in a beautiful fountain, notice the light making rainbows shimmer and dance among the droplets of water. Let the pain flow out from you down through your feet along with the rivulets of water. Feel your body and spirit become free, alive, and invigorated by the sparkling water.*

or

> *You see a flowing, bubbling stream with sunlight sparkling on the glistening pebbles as the water tumbles and rushes over them. You are drawn to the stream and sit on the bank with your feet in the cool water. You feel the relief as the water soothes and relaxes you, and any painful sensations drain from your body, downstream and out to the sea.*

or

*Lie down in a warm, blue healing pool. It could be on the beach or a marble pool indoors. Let the soothing blueness envelop you and permeate right through your body to release anything you don't need, such as any pain or unwanted emotion. Let it all float out and away from you. Feel yourself soothed and cradled by the blue, blue water.*

*When you have spent enough time with the water image of your choice, complete the visualization by gradually coming back to the room, taking the feelings of peace and freedom with you.*

These images and any others involving water, such as standing in a waterfall or an effervescent spring, floating in the sea or taking a foamy bubble bath, are truly relaxing and pain-relieving. As always when using visualization, go deeply into the scene and let yourself see and sense everything about the place you are in, experiencing it fully.

## Change the Pain Visualization

One of the most effective ways of all to reduce pain is to use visualization techniques to obtain an image of the pain itself and then change it to one more tolerable, or even make the pain disappear altogether. When you are in a relaxed mode and your imaginative, creative mind is freed, you are able to allow spontaneous images or symbols into your mind of how the pain seems to look or feel. You can then use your imaginative skills to work with the pain symbols to change them. You can loosen tight sensations, cool down hot areas, and soften stabbing sensations. Trust your imaginative mind and accept the symbols and images that come to you first, as these will be the true impression you have of your pain and therefore the most effective with which to work.

When you begin this kind of creative visualization, it is best if you start with relaxing your body and mind with your Safe Haven Visualization. Once you are completely relaxed, you can allow spontaneous images of your pain to come to your mind and thus be in the right receptive mood to begin work on them.

*As always, find a quiet, comfortable place where you may be at peace for a short while. Close your eyes and pay attention to your breathing . . . let it be quiet and relaxed. . . . Allow your body to become still. . . . Feel relaxation begin to spread throughout your body . . . just let everything go. . . . When thoughts come into your mind, let them go too. . . . Enjoy the peace and comfort you have created. . . . And now take your mind to your safe haven. . . . This is your very own special place, a space where you are able to feel totally at one with yourself and the world. . . . Travel in your mind around your haven. See, feel, hear everything about it . . . enjoy being there. Spend as long as you want in this place.*

*Now that you are relaxed, peaceful, and calm, know that the healing process has already begun. Keep breathing naturally and easily as you approach in your mind the area with which you want to work. Don't do anything; just keep breathing gently and allow the pain to come to the forefront of your consciousness. Be open and receptive and willing to allow the pain itself to suggest images to you. Ask yourself, "What is the pain, or sensation, like?" Take note of the very first images that flash into your mind or sensations you feel in your body. These will be the most important upon which to work. Keep breathing quietly and just allow the pain to be there. There's no need to try to find something and no need to shift around or to move anything. Simply be passive and allow sensations to come to you without judging them or reacting in any way.*

*The information may come as:*

*A fleeting picture in your mind*
*A color, shape, or texture*
*A vague sensation or feeling inside yourself*
*A physical sensation*
*A sound or a voice*
*A taste*
*Simply "knowing" something*

*When you sleep, you may have images of your pain in your dreams. If so, it is a good idea to use those images as starting points as your subconscious mind has already produced them for you.*

What you receive will be a symbol of how your subconscious mind views the pain. Whatever you see, hear, or feel is right for *you*. Sometimes you may have not an image but a general sensation such as tightness or soreness. If this is the case, to clarify the sensation, ask yourself: "What sort of tightness?" "What is the soreness like?" or "What does this remind me of?" Never judge what arrives in your mind. Leave your critical and logical left-brain faculties behind—you are tapping into the creative right side of your brain. Whatever springs into your imagination is coming from you and so is perfect for the occasion—trust your intuitive self. Don't rush the process; relax and accept whatever comes. If nothing comes, place your attention on your breathing and spend more time continuing to relax. The imaginative process cannot be *made* to operate, and needs a relaxed mind and attitude to flourish.

Continue with further questions in order to gather as much information as you can in order to gain a clear picture. The more information you have, the more successful you can be when finding images to alter the pain sensations.

*Ask yourself questions about the size of the image . . . the color . . . the shape. . . . Does it change or is the image constant? . . . Are there any associated sounds, smells, or tastes to the pain? . . . Is it hot or cold? . . . Are there any memories associated with it? . . . Is it trying to tell you something? . . . Are there any emotions or feelings associated with it? . . . How do you feel toward it? . . . Does it remind you of anything?*

When you first use this process, you may well receive a faint glimmer or flicker of an image or sensation. With practice, as you continue to use the process, the images will become stronger and more detailed. Remember not to force or strain for images; allow them to arise by themselves. If you find that you are beginning to *try*, take your mind away, either to your breath or to your haven. Often, as soon as you go "off watch" and relax, an image will present itself. Remember to use the first image that comes to your mind, no matter what it is.

Don't worry if nothing comes and you don't notice anything: just continue to breathe quietly and normally for a little while longer. Be nonjudgmental about yourself and about the process.

> *When you have as full an image as you are able to at this time, you can begin to change it, alter it, and finally release it.*
>
> *Make this vital part of your visualization really strong and powerful—the stronger the new image, the more effective it will be. The altered image may be humorous or even ridiculous, it doesn't matter; often, in fact, these may be the most effective, as you will have injected emotion into the process. In your mind, gradually change heat into coolness, change a fiery red into a calming blue, loosen and undo a tight band, smooth out a crumpled part with an iron, extinguish flames with foam or water, imagine healing golden light soothing sore areas, soften iron bars as though they are ice or ice cream melting or turn them to spongy rubber, loosen off a tight area . . . be inventive. Spend some time visualizing the image changing until the sensations lessen and your body is more comfortable.*

A successful visualization of mine was to change a headache that seemed like a tight band around my head into a coronet of blue forget-me-nots just above my head. My headache disappeared and I spent a whole day with my invisible "halo" because I enjoyed the pleasurable sensations of freedom I gained about my neck, shoulders, and head.

You could continue by asking the painful area if there is anything you can do to help it. Again, don't expect an answer; just be open to anything that comes to your mind. Answers may be elusive if you search too hard. Have, instead, an attitude of watching and observing. You may have a sense that you could soothe your pain with massage, or that it needs cool water or a comforting hot-water bottle. Whatever it is, imagine giving yourself what the pain needs, perhaps massaging in a soothing oil, taking a natural pain-relief concoction of soothing syrup, standing in a hot shower, lying under a healing lamp, lying on warm sand on a beach . . . use the creative side of your mind.

Occasionally you may have a picture or sensation you don't understand. Don't dismiss it: put it to one side and possibly later on in the day you may realize what it meant. You can then deal with it as necessary.

> *Last, visualize all the joys of being free from pain . . . being healthy . . . comfortable . . . and strong. . . . Find an image that appeals to you to represent your body's natural painkillers, the endorphins, as they flow throughout your body . . . perhaps shooting stars, silver arrows, golden light, or soothing pink oil. . . . Make this a really strong image that you can use often. . . . See yourself happy . . . laughing . . . and moving freely. . . . See yourself getting better and better every day . . . and know you have achieved this by yourself with your own natural powers. . . . Congratulate yourself on dealing so well with your pain . . . feel proud of yourself. . . . Make sure you see your success really strongly and clearly.*
>
> *When you have completed this last part of the visualization, lie quietly for a moment or two until you are ready to begin movement again . . . then, slowly and gently return to the room, feeling relaxed and full of well-being, knowing what you have done and learned is of value.*

The more experience you have with changing your pain images in this way, the more effective the process will become. Some people may gain success with Change the Pain very quickly, others need lots of practice: so be patient and keep practicing. Later on, when you have had more practice and feel confident about approaching your pain in this way, you may find you can obtain images very quickly, without a long relaxation session first. Some people are able instantly to reach down inside themselves to receive information. This does require total ease with getting in touch with your intuitive self.

It is often helpful to draw a picture of your pain image and another one of how you altered it. Have a pencil and paper ready beside you so you can jot down lines while the images are fresh in your mind. Make sure the altered image is really strong and clear. The drawing need be just a very rough outline and it is for your eyes only, so feel free to make it as loose and unsophisticated as you like.

To summarize the Change the Pain Visualization, remember to cover all the following points:

1. Relax your body.
2. Relax your mind with your Safe Haven Visualization.
3. Allow an image of the pain to surface in your mind.
4. Change the image to another that is more agreeable.
5. Ask the pain if you can help it in any way.
6. Visualize being fit and healthy, moving easily and with comfort.

### Two-Minute Healing Visualization

To reinforce our other healing and pain-relieving visualizations, there follows a quick, two-minute healing experience. Use this powerful visualization at least three times every day for intensive "bursts" of healing and see what a difference it will make to how you feel. Every time you open your mind in this way, you also allow all the cells of your body to function normally and facilitate and smooth the path of your natural healing processes.

> *This time, you need not be sitting or lying down. This visualization may be used wherever you are; tailor it to the situation in which you find yourself. Just* STOP *whatever you are doing and mentally withdraw into yourself and concentrate on your breath as it flows in and out of your body. Allow your breathing to be natural and quiet. Be aware that you now feel relaxed, calm, and centered.*
>
> *Imagine you are holding your cupped hands up to the sun, the source of all life. In your imagination, feel its energy and warmth on your hands and face. (If you want, and you are in a convenient place to do so, you may raise your hands in reality as though to the sun. You will, with awareness, feel energy tingling in your fingers, which can then be brought down, very gently, in your cupped hands to your abdomen, where your hands can rest awhile.)*

*Whether in imagination or reality, feel the energy and warmth moving along your arms and all around your body. See the energy as a beautiful soft golden healing light . . . let it flow all around your body . . . see it concentrating in the parts needing extra soothing and healing. . . . Imagine the golden light filling your whole body. . . . Imagine there is so much light that it overflows and moves outward to surround you like a lovely glowing golden aura all around your body, as though you are in a shining capsule of healing light. . . . Really have a sense of being cradled in this golden light, feel protected and joyful. Now say an uplifting affirmation to yourself, such as "Every cell in my body is healthy and strong." When it is time to bring your visualization to an end, return to your breathing for a few moments and know that healing is taking place.*

Make a date with yourself to use the Two-Minute Healing at least three times a day, more if possible. Do it in the bath, on a train, while waiting for an appointment, or at any other spare moment. You don't even have to shut your eyes and so no one would guess what you are doing. The more often you consciously get in touch with yourself in this way, the easier it is for your healing processes to function efficiently and normally. Speak to and encourage your billions of cells; they thrive in a joyful, happy, and confident body.

## USING VISUALIZATION SKILLS

Once we are familiar with the visualization technique, we can be adventurous and use our new skills even more creatively. Visualization is excellent for rehearsing coming events in our imagination to give us a clear picture of how we will perform on the actual occasion. It can be useful for running through how we will handle, say, an important meeting, a visit from relations, a consultation with the doctor, or a journey. We can use the process for lifestyle changes, such as losing weight, enjoying peaceful sleep at night, and moving to a new home. We can contact our intuition and work with it, using as its symbol an imaginary inner friend or wise counselor.

All of these types of visualizations lead to a greater depth of knowledge and understanding about ourselves. We get in touch with the part of us that is deeply intuitive and knows what is best for us, perhaps asking simple, or even profound, questions and receiving real answers as we become more and more in touch with our innermost feelings. We grow as a person and find that natural pain relief and healing follow automatically when we use our innate abilities in this caring way.

## ACTION GUIDELINES

1. Practice the basic skills of visualization at every possible opportunity and listen to the CD that accompanies this book.
2. Develop your own Safe Haven Visualization, using all your senses to make your peaceful inner space as familiar to you as your everyday surroundings. Use your safe haven as often as you can. It is a life-enhancing place where you can be refreshed and uplifted.
3. Use your Safe Haven Visualization as a starting point for other visualizations, such as fantasy adventures, healing and pain relief, goal setting such as walking and sitting improvement, boosting self-esteem, rehearsal of future events, exploration of emotions and situations, and contacting and consulting personal inner guides.
4. Use positive statements (affirmations) to reinforce visualizations. These two techniques together are highly effective.
5. If a pain flare-up occurs, use creative visualization and affirmations to ease the path toward healing.
6. If you are having treatment of some kind, use positive visualization to reinforce the success of the treatment.
7. Picture yourself always as being full of radiant health; hold this image near to you, whatever your condition. Our natural healing process is greatly enhanced with a positive attitude supported by creative visualization and affirmations.

# UNIT 5
■
# Dealing With
# Your Feelings

**CONTENTS**

# Dealing With Your Feelings

## YOUR EMOTIONAL LIFE

Our feelings are constantly changing. When we are happy, loving, and full of gratitude for life, we feel in touch with ourselves, at one with the world, and life seems to flow. These positive feelings are normal and natural for us. When we have negative feelings, such as anger and fear, we often feel out of touch or uncomfortable with ourselves, everything may appear to be against us, and life seems blocked and difficult. It is also perfectly normal and natural to have these negative feelings. However, it is important that we have strategies to express our negative feelings and maintain a harmony with the world. It becomes even more important when we have pain in our lives, because just as muscle tension can create pain or worsen the severity of pain, so emotional tension can affect our pain. The state of our emotions has a direct bearing on our physical body. For example, if we are feeling happy, our muscles relax; if we are feeling tense and irritable, they tighten. Therefore, it makes sense that by being able to release emotional tension, we can often also release muscular tension, thus reducing pain.

When we have pain, our feelings tend to be heightened because of the additional pressure from our physical sensations. We can be subject to a whole range of negative feelings, and our view of our situation and of the world as a whole can become distorted and out of perspective. Rational, constructive thought is not available to us, nothing seems to flow, and we cannot see our way through to calm waters. This is a common reaction with pain and perfectly understandable; it is reassuring to know there is nothing wrong, bad, or abnormal in any of these feelings, as it is impossible for anyone to have only positive feelings the whole time. Any way you feel, any emotion, is perfectly normal, and so don't criticize yourself if you feel angry about your pain or fearful that a flare-up won't settle. When we have pain, we cope the best we know how at the time. This unit will show you new ways of dealing with unwanted negative emotions.

Although there are no "wrong" or "bad" ways to *feel*, there are definitely inappropriate ways to *express* the feelings. For example, we may slam down crockery and utensils in the kitchen when our anger is not with the utensils or having to make a meal, but instead, in reality, with the pain. Other people cope by appearing to be completely in control, but they may, in fact, be hiding their feelings. However, this repression of emotions aggravates the situation: the emotions don't go away; they remain inside. Concealment of feelings, or the failure to acknowledge emotions and to express them in an appropriate way, can cause a buildup of tension within us. This tension can sap our energy—and we need that energy to take care of ourselves. As Professor Jon Kabat-Zinn, of the University of Massachusetts, says in his book *Full Catastrophe Living,* "Our emotional pain . . . is a messenger. Feelings have to be acknowledged. If we ignore them or repress them or suppress them or sublimate them, they fester and yield no resolution, no peace."

In addition to acknowledging our feelings and expressing them, we need to handle the situation that sparked off the feeling and find out if there are any practical actions we could take to help to solve the problem at its root. Often problems become obscured by our strong feelings about them, leaving us unable to think clearly and rationally about the solution. Therefore, any action we take may not truly be to our best advantage. For instance, we may take rash action in the heat of the moment, when perhaps a more measured approach would have been preferable.

Using the techniques in this unit will enable you to deal with emotional turmoil or extremes of feelings in a positive manner so you may return to emotional balance and harmony. The techniques will show you how to tap in to your own natural inner resources and wisdom, helping to release unwanted feelings and to solve the problem that gave rise to the feelings. This innate wisdom is your deepest and most abiding natural inner strength. This wisdom is always there, available to you, and always will be there, even in the depths of despair or the height of anger—if only you can take a moment to call upon it. You can learn to face your negative feelings and release them once and for all.

## RESPONDING TO EMOTIONAL SITUATIONS

We can learn to deal more effectively with some emotional situations so that we side-step excessive emotional upheaval. It has to be accepted, though, that our emotions *are* changeable and we cannot expect to reach a stage when we never feel some emotional pain; it is just not humanly possible. However, we *can* learn better ways of dealing with some potentially distressing situations to defuse the situation or moderate the effects.

Always remember, it isn't the other person or situation that has upset us: we have upset ourselves—we make ourselves angry, anxious, or upset by our response. By realizing we have upset ourselves and that it is not someone else's fault, we become more in control of the situation. We are responsible for the way we feel, and we can work on handling our own emotions. We cannot change other people and the way they think or act; we can only change ourselves.

When you are feeling ill at ease, you may notice some of the following sensations: a tightening in your body, tingling in your legs, feelings of pressure in your chest, anxious thoughts, feeling hot and/or flushing, your heart beating faster, or a dry mouth. If you are stressed, even slightly, your body becomes aroused and ready to either run away or stay and fight. This would have worked fine if you were confronted with an attack in the Stone Age, but these days you aren't normally faced with a woolly mammoth! The Stone Age person's body would become prepared to either flee or stay and fight by sending surges of adrenaline into the system and by moving blood to the arm and leg muscles for strength and to the brain to facilitate quick thinking. After the exertion of either fighting or running away, the body would rapidly return to normal and the episode would be forgotten. These symptoms are known as the "fight-or-flight" reactions.

These days, instead of facing woolly mammoths, we may have to deal with the doctor, a relation, or even our own thoughts. The body doesn't know the difference between a really threatening situation and an imagined one, and so any surge of fear readies it to fight or run. Of course, in our society, we often can't do either of those things and thus we stifle our natural reactions and emotions. When we do this, instead of the adrenaline being used to enable us to either fight or run away, it remains with us and disperses slowly, and we feel some or all of the anxiety symptoms. All of which, of course, makes the whole event even more stressful and painful.

We have learned already that when faced with an uncomfortable situation, we tend to react to it in a habitual way learned a long time ago. Often we do this by suppressing our feelings or acting hastily and thereby perhaps aggravating the whole event. If, instead, as soon as we notice that we are beginning to feel uncomfortable in a situation we can take a moment to use the next technique, we can then choose our response in a calmer fashion. The method is simple, but it does take a lot of practice to learn to become aware of what is happening and to intervene in time, before feelings get out of hand. Try it for yourself. If you manage to respond in a calmer fashion just once, it will give you the experience and confidence to know you can achieve it again. Gradually you will be able to take charge in more of the potentially emotional situations you encounter.

## THE "STOP" TECHNIQUE

The "STOP" technique will teach you how to prevent the emotional situation from escalating, or to accept and deal with the emotions if they do develop.

*When you sense that you are just beginning to feel unease in a situation, face it by saying to yourself, inside your head,*

"STOP"

*and immediately concentrate on your breathing. Now you are in control again, albeit for a moment.*

*Maintain the advantage of being in control by swiftly taking your attention to your abdomen and allowing your breath to become slower and deeper. This takes only a split second and will give you a break from the potentially stressful situation. It will allow you mentally to stand back slightly, rather like an observer of the situation, enabling you to respond in a more rational way rather than reacting automatically. Tell yourself* "Stay calm" *or* "I can cope with this" *while you think what your response will be.*

*Remember:* Don't fight or try to suppress the uneasy feelings; this adds tension. Concentrate instead on your actions or tactics. Try to keep some of your attention on your breath as the situation develops.

You will find that by standing back a little from the situation, you won't become sucked into escalating emotions so easily; this will enable you to respond more effectively.

## FEELING THE FEELINGS

If, after saying STOP, you do become taken over by an emotion, know that you can still handle the experience effectively by facing and feeling the force of the feelings, becoming totally aware of the whole emotion: "I am feeling bad today," "I am feeling so sad," "I am feeling anxious and panicky," or whatever is the emotion.

*Knowing* just what it is we are feeling is healing in itself. By allowing ourselves to accept and live the emotion fully, with total awareness, we can ride it out. The emotion may still affect us, but we will not be so completely in its grip. We may even be able to think, if somewhat ruefully, "What a lot of pain and suffering I can cause myself!" We will gain from knowing that the emotional wave and the physical reactions will rise, peak, and fall away again into calm on the other side. The emotion and the physical reactions *will* pass—they always do.

This total mindfulness and acceptance of the emotion and the physical reactions will generate feelings of kindliness and compassion toward ourselves as we grow to understand that our emotions *will* pass and we *can* cope. We are *more* than our emotions, *more* than our pain. Concentrating on maintaining slow diaphragmatic breathing during the period of heightened emotions will help to calm and relax us as we go with the emotions.

The technique for coping with extremes of feelings can be summed up simply as follows:

STOP and . . .
*Face,* don't fight the feeling.
*Accept* and *allow* the physical and emotional reactions.
*Watch* and *wait,* as an observer.
*Concentrate* on deep, abdominal (diaphragmatic) breathing.
*Know* that the feelings and sensations will pass.

We may find that there's an element of "I wish I hadn't done/said that" within the emotion. Peace will come when we can accept that the past is over and done with and cannot be changed. Peace will come when we can accept what is present, or has happened, as it *is*, without rejecting, judging, or wanting to alter it in any way. Acceptance doesn't mean we either *like* the situation or are resigned to it, but that we accept that the occurrence, whatever it is, has happened; it is a fact that cannot be altered and the only way out is to move on and begin afresh. This kind of accepting attitude can take time to grow, but life is so much easier for us when we allow it to happen, and we can help its progress with the above technique of total mindfulness of the emotion, fully feeling the feeling.

## SEEKING UNDERSTANDING WITHIN

Actions or decisions taken at times of heightened emotions tend to be colored by our emotional reasoning or reactions, rather than coming from our inner wisdom, and so we are better advised to wait until we can access that wiser part of ourselves before we act. This knowledge in itself can be of comfort if we are emotionally distressed. We will understand that the emotion will pass and that action can wait until we are feeling calmer.

It's not always possible to stop and use a technique when emotions are heightened, and the following Seeking Understanding Within technique can be used afterward to help sort out your feelings when you feel stuck in an emotional situation. Use the technique as often as you feel you need to; it is of great value in understanding your emotional life, helping you to focus inwardly and to see the problem with clarity, allowing your natural wisdom to come to the fore. Practicing the technique will give you strength in the future when dealing with heightened emotions. With the technique you can think and write what you honestly feel, no holds barred. The Seeking Understanding Within technique is designed for you to:

- Accept your emotion by naming it. Acknowledging and taking responsibility for your emotions is the beginning of the healing process.
- Open yourself to any messages coming from the emotion.
- Uncover the teaching within the emotion that will give you freedom from it. This step handles the emotion in a practical way and may involve taking some action.

## How to Use the Technique

*Take five or ten minutes for yourself and make yourself comfortable, with paper and pencil at hand. Use the technique with a relaxed, open mind with an attitude of compassion and loving-kindness toward yourself.*

*Place your attention on your breath and follow it with your mind for a few moments, allowing it to become a little slower and deeper. Allow yourself to relax; feel safe and secure.*

### 1. Identifying the Emotion

*Draw a circle at the top of a page. In the middle of the circle write down the emotional upset. Identify it as clearly as you can; be specific—for example, "I feel angry" or "I feel anxious" or "I feel sad" . . . or whatever is your own emotional concern.*

*Example:*

I feel angry

## 2. Recognizing the Messages from the Emotion

*Look at your words in the circle. This will focus your mind and allow your real thoughts to come to the surface. As a thought comes to you, draw a short line from the circle and write the thought next to it. Approach the exercise with an open mind and open heart. There's no need to try to find thoughts or to strain for them; just let them arise spontaneously. Always, always take note of the first thoughts that appear in your mind, no matter how trivial or unimportant they may seem at the time.*

*Keep repeating "I feel . . . [the emotion]" in between each thought you write, jotting down the new thoughts as they come, and continuing until no more thoughts arise. These are the thoughts behind the emotion. This is what you are telling yourself and what you are really feeling. Although you may be surprised at some of the thoughts that come to you, just accept them. You may find that you uncover some deep truths about your feelings.*

## 3. Understanding the Emotion

*Write the question below on your piece of paper underneath your jotted thoughts above.*

*"What is it about my feeling that I need to understand?"*

*Look at your circle and the thoughts you have written around it and ask yourself the question. As you ask the question, open your mind and be receptive to any thoughts that come to you. Trust your intuition; you are not "thinking" with your logical mind about the emotion but rather allowing your inner wisdom to surface. Write down the very first thought or feeling that comes to you,* whatever it is. *This time, write your thoughts straight down the page underneath the question. Then ask yourself the question again and write down the very next thought. Continue to repeat the question and jot down each thought arising in response to the question. Be totally honest and write down all the thoughts, no matter what they are. Keep going until no more thoughts about the question surface.*

*These messages will give you understanding about the emotion you are feeling. The emotion, although it may be upsetting, is a teacher for you. You will learn from the emotion and perhaps understand more about yourself and gain insight into how you "work" emotionally. When we ask ourselves questions with a noncritical, nonjudgmental, non-skeptical attitude and with a relaxed kindness and compassion, allowing ourselves to be open to any answers, without forcing or straining for them, wonders happen—we become tuned in to our own natural inner self, which will give us wise answers. We do know, deep inside us, what is best for us and what the truth is for us about particular situations. We can help ourselves: the answers are inside us all along.*

## 4. Gaining Freedom from the Emotion

*This stage teaches you how to release an emotional block. Write the following question and then note down your answers as they come to you.*

*"What can I learn from all of this that will release me from the emotion?"*

*Again, approach the question with an open attitude, allowing answers to arise spontaneously. Remember to write down the very first thoughts appearing in your mind.*

*Continue like this, asking the question and writing down each thought. Keep going until you feel better. You may suddenly have a feeling of "That's it" or "I understand." This will tell you that you have the answer. It may take the form of a feeling of lightness inside you, as though a bright light has been switched on around the situation. You will know with certainty that you have the answer and need go no further.*

## 5. Accepting the Situation

*The final question to ask is:*

*"Is there any action I could take?"*

*When asking "Is there any action . . ." you may realize that there is none; but that will be a satisfactory answer in itself. Some situations need to be accepted just as they are. We cannot always find something to be done in a particular situation, other than accept it as it is.*

## 6. Thanking Your Inner Wisdom for Its Help

*A last step, which it is very important to take, is to thank your inner wisdom for helping you. The more you praise your inner abilities, the better you will feel and the more likely you are to get closer to your natural inner self on another occasion. You are developing a relationship with your wise inner self and, like all relationships, it needs to be nurtured. After all, it is you whom you are praising, and we can all do with as much praise and encouragement as possible—we can never receive too much. We thrive on praise and need to know that we approve of ourselves. We flourish and grow in a support-ive, encouraging atmosphere where we know we are worthy of value and respected, especially by ourselves. If you find this rather embarrassing or difficult at first, a good way to thank yourself is to imagine that you are expressing your gratitude to a wise old friend.*

*If you discovered that there is some action to take, make sure you take your own good advice and use the information gained to plan how to carry out the action.*

# HOW TO SAY WHAT YOU FEEL—WITHOUT PROVOKING AN ARGUMENT

Everyday communication with other people can be difficult enough at the best of times, and when we have chronic pain, it is even more important that we learn how to communicate our feelings well. It may sound obvious, but *unless we say what it is we want or feel, no one will know!* We often *assume* people understand what we are trying to say to them, expecting them to somehow know or guess what it is we are really saying or want.

We may then be surprised, hurt, or angry when the other person doesn't respond as we wish. Often people speak to each other with a hidden "code" or meaning; they say one thing but mean another. This makes life very difficult and can lead to arguments and misunderstandings.

In order to have our needs met, we have to be able to tell others exactly what it is we want in a plain, simple, and straightforward manner. There is a knack or skill to this that will make life much easier for everyone concerned.

> *When trying to let it be known how you are feeling, always start with an "I" statement and identify your emotion: for example, "I feel really upset because . . ." If, instead, you say, "You make me upset when you . . ." this puts the other person on the defensive and the result is far more likely to be one of ill-feeling.*

This straightforward way of saying what you feel or want works very well because the other person understands what you are saying without being threatened by it in any way.

## OTHER WAYS TO DEAL WITH EMOTIONS

There may be times when we feel it is not appropriate to use the previous techniques, and on those occasions we can use some of the following alternative approaches to relieve emotional tension. We know that physical activity often shifts negative emotions, but if we are in pain, we may not be able to go for a bracing walk in the country or chop up a pile of wood. We can, however, find other ways to dispel pent-up feelings and to change our mood.

An excellent way to release our feelings, whatever they may be, is to *write* them out of our system. Sometimes we don't really know what it is that is making us feel upset; we may *think* we know but often there is something deeper behind the actual situation that provoked an emotional response. Bringing emotions out into the open is a healing process in itself; the emotional energy is released and no longer rules our behavior. The physical activity of writing contributes to the release.

## Write It Away

When we are writing in this next exercise, we are not *thinking* about the emotion. Thinking about it, going over and over it, or analyzing it, will never make an emotion disappear—feelings are for *feeling*, not thinking about. We are going to experience the feeling and, by physically expressing it onto paper, release it. It is particularly good to use this technique when we are in the midst of emotional turmoil. As in the previous technique where we contacted our inner wisdom, we are getting in touch with our natural *feeling* self, not our intellectual self.

You will need paper and a ballpoint pen or a supply of pencils.

1. *Make sure you have a space for yourself where you won't be interrupted when you are in full writing flow. Make sure you are in a comfortable position for writing. Relax a little by becoming aware of your breath as it flows in and out. Notice the slight movements of your lower ribs and abdomen as you inhale and exhale, and allow your breathing to become a little slower and deeper.*

2. *Now recall the event that triggered the particular emotion you want to deal with—anger, fear, envy, or whatever. Visualize the occasion as vividly as you can, with as much detail as possible, until you feel you are in contact with the emotional response to that event. When you are in touch with the emotion, you may feel it as physical sensations in your body: a tightening or "butterflies-in-the-stomach" sensation or feelings of pressure or heat in, possibly, your stomach, chest, face, or throat area.*

3. *You can now express the emotion through your writing so it can*

*be dispelled in a safe way, without harming or confronting anyone. Write down any thought that comes to you. Don't censor anything, no matter how silly or "unthinkable" the thoughts are; allow yourself to really let rip. Just get those feelings out. You may find yourself crying or talking out loud as the feelings become stronger. That's good; keep going and write out any anxieties and anger. It may be about some everyday matter or it may be about your pain or any other subject. If it's about the pain, write down any thoughts and fears about coping with the pain, any fears about whether it will go away again, perhaps anger at your medical treatment, about your job and, yes, even your anger at your family. Write down all those thoughts you daren't normally express—let them pour out. This is the place to get rid of them. Don't worry if you break your pencil point as you let out your frustrations; pick up another pencil and carry on.*

4. *Don't look back at what you have written, just keep on writing. You will probably find you write faster and faster, especially if the emotion you are feeling is anger. You can rant and swear on the paper: it doesn't matter, no one else will see it, no one will criticize you. Let spelling, grammar, or any other normal writing considerations go out of the window; you can leave sentences unfinished if the thoughts come too fast to write down. Don't read it through. Just write.*

5. *Keep writing until you feel peaceful and free from the emotion. You will know when the emotion is spent.*

6. *Now that you are feeling calmer, destroy the paper without reading it. Tear it into tiny pieces or burn it safely, but don't read it through.*

7. *As always,* thank and praise yourself *for releasing the emotion in this way.*

As you do this exercise, you may discover all kinds of truths about what you really feel, things you may have been hiding even from yourself. Once they are in the open, you are free of them and, if there is any action required, you can deal with it rationally and positively. Understanding your emotions is crucial to becoming at ease with them. A friend who had a pain flare-up did this exercise when she was really angry and upset at not being able to attend a long-standing engagement. After the writing exercise, she found that she had uncovered a deep fear of being left alone, unable to cope by herself. She could then tackle that issue and work out how she could cope in such a situation. She felt reassured and much more secure afterward. She no longer felt so angry once she understood the fears behind her anger. Now, in similar situations, she is able to think to herself, "Oh, here I go again! I am coping perfectly well and I always will find ways of coping. Now I will concentrate on what I *can* do."

As you express your frustrations and fears on paper with this exercise, you become free of them. Use it often.

## Using the Power of the Imagination to Dispel Unwanted Emotions

The next few simple techniques use the power of your imagination to shift unwanted feelings. When you use your imagination in the following ways, make sure you have a few quiet moments to yourself where you can be undisturbed. Sit or lie as comfortably as you can and, by placing your attention on your abdomen for a few moments, allow your breathing to become slower and deeper before you start.

### The River

*Imagine all the unwanted emotional energy moving out from you and into your hand, where you condense it into a stone. Feel the sensation of the stone in your hand for a moment and then, in your imagination, throw it away from you as hard as you can into a river, where it will be washed clean of the unwanted feelings. Imagine how the emotions will dissolve and, like mud, will be swept out to sea and diluted where they can harm no one. Enjoy the relief.*

### Visualizing Physical Activities

If we were completely fit, we could safely disperse negative emotional energy by jumping up and down in a fury, laying into a punching bag, or giving ourselves a full body shake. Those of us for whom such dramatic physical exertions are not possible or advisable can use the visualization of energetic physical activity as a substitute for actual physical activity in changing a mood. If you cannot chop up that pile of wood or go for a bracing walk, visualize doing so in full detail, really feeling all the physical movements and sensations. Create a whole picture in your mind with as much detail as you can of the sights and sounds involved. For example:

> *Visualize yourself outside on a bright autumn day. There is a pile of logs in front of you. See and feel the texture of a log as you pick it up and place it on top of another flat log. In your hand you have an ax. Feel the weight of the ax. Measure up the log with your eye, swing the ax down and behind you and then bring it up high and over onto the top log. Watch it split satisfyingly into two. Continue doing this until you have a whole pile of neatly stacked logs ready for your fire.*

or

> *Use your imagination to see all your emotional worries and problems turning into leaves. Imagine that you are sweeping the leaves vigorously away with a big garden broom. Feel a strong wind blowing around you that picks up the leaves and takes them far away, out of sight.*

## Brushing Off Unwanted Negative Energies

We can also dispel unwanted negativity by "brushing" it off.

> *Start with your face, placing one hand on either side of your forehead, your palms toward your face, not quite touching your skin. Now brush off the feelings, giving a slight flick with your fingers at the end of each stroke, as though you are brushing away mist or smoke. Brush and flick away those feelings around your face, from under your chin and throat, then up and away from your forehead and the back of your head. You can sometimes touch yourself, sometimes not; it doesn't matter. You can then do the same for your whole body, or as much of it as you can reach: out from the center of your chest, across each shoulder and arm, and so on right down your body, as far as you can reach, finishing*

*with your toes, flicking away the last vestige of negativity. If you can't reach your toes, brush in the air in the general direction of your feet. You may find that you feel as though some areas need more brushing than others. When you have flicked and brushed away the feelings, you might like to soothe yourself in the following way.*

## Soothing Yourself

*This time, as you go around your body, smooth yourself down, as though you were stroking ruffled feathers or fur, sometimes touching your body, sometimes not touching. Start around your face and head and work your way down as far as you can reach. Afterward, sit still for a few moments, letting your feet sink down into the ground. Enjoy the calmer feelings you will now have.*

## A Magic Capsule

If you find you have difficulty in handling a particular situation or person, you may want to try protecting yourself from his or her influence using the powers of your imagination in the following way.

*Imagine you are surrounded with an aura of golden light. In your imagination, let the light flow all around you so if anyone could see it, you would appear to be in a beautiful golden capsule. Now imagine that the outer surface of the magic golden capsule hardens and toughens so it forms a thick, impenetrable barrier between you and the person or situation that is potentially disturbing to you. See yourself as being mentally and emotionally powerful and strong inside your shell. Know that nothing, no words, no action, can harm you. You can say to yourself, "I am strong and protected" or "I am the power in my life." Choose words with which you are comfortable yourself. See yourself smiling, strong and invincible, unaffected by any situation in which you find yourself.*

Try this method and see if you can maintain your magic capsule during a difficult situation. Choose a situation that is not too threatening to start with, while you are still developing your imagination. Like most skills, this Magic Capsule technique will become more and more effective with practice.

## A Cloak of Invincibility

A variation on the same theme as the Magic Capsule is the Cloak of Invincibility.

> *Wear your Cloak of Invincibility at times of stress. Imagine you have a special cloak. It could be gold or silver or a midnight blue full-length velvet cloak with silver spangles upon it—you choose your own special protective robe. Imagine that once you don this cloak, it protects you from outside influences and you feel safe and powerful inside it.*

This is another mental device, a mental "trick," but it doesn't matter. If it works for you—*use it.* Be receptive to new ideas and give them a chance.

## Grounding Yourself

When you find yourself becoming carried away with any kind of feeling and need to take control again, come down to earth—literally. Practice the following earthing or grounding exercise to bring you back into your own calm domain where *you* are in charge. By grounding yourself, you reconnect with the earth or surface under your feet; you then become calmer and regain your sense of yourself.

> *Either sitting or standing, place your feet flat on the floor or earth. Let your weight sink down through your feet into the ground. Move your weight about a little, backward and forward and from side to side, so you feel real contact with the floor or earth before you come to stillness. Make sure your toes are uncurled and your weight is slightly heavier going through your heels. When you are still, become aware of more and more contact with the ground.*
>
> *Let your weight sink right into the ground. You are reconnecting yourself with the earth; you are becoming part of the*

*earth itself, like an old oak tree with its strong roots going deep into the ground, anchoring you into the very earth itself. Like the oak tree, you are strengthened and nourished by the earth. Storms may break all around the oak tree but it sits firmly and is unaffected. You feel totally secure with your place in life and full of a wonderful sense of belonging with the whole of nature.*

Practice this exercise by yourself at first and then see if you can maintain your sense of being firmly grounded when you are with other people or are feeling emotionally upset, in pain, or tired. It will help you to stay calm, in touch with yourself, and in control.

## FOSTERING POSITIVE EMOTIONS

Most of the emphasis in this unit has been on negative emotions. The unit would not be complete if it did not mention our positive emotions. When we have pain in our lives, we may feel these positive emotions less often than before, but we can do much to foster and encourage them. So, savor those tiny moments of pleasure, make the most of them, expand them; don't let them slip away almost unnoticed. We can only benefit from maximizing every ounce of enjoyment we can find in our lives.

### *Maximize the Moment*

1. *Try to become more aware of when you are feeling pleased, happy, generous, thankful, amused, or any other positive emotion. Note what it was that made you respond in a positive way—and see if you can repeat the event giving rise to the emotion.*

2. *When you do notice a fleeting feeling of pleasure—when, say, completing a minor task such as the washing up,* maximize it by *really noticing what you are doing: see the sparkle on the dishes, the neat pile of plates, the shining cutlery, the clean pans,* be pleased with yourself. *Don't underestimate the power of these brief moments of pleasure; they add up to a totally different attitude to life.*

3. *Read Unit 8, entitled Enjoying Yourself, and make sure you find at least one occasion in every day when you actively enjoy yourself, even if it is something very simple.*

4. *Do something creative every day. When we are being creative, we are fully in touch with our inner wisdom and powers. We feel fully involved, happy, and content. It doesn't matter what it is you are doing, only that your attention is fully engaged using the creative power of your mind.*

5. *Be sensational! Indulge your senses. Enjoy your favorite food, drink, sights, fragrances, and touch sensations. Include them in "set pieces" of pleasure. Plan to have special "sense sessions" in which every sense is catered to. Choose a favorite time of your own and plan to enjoy it to the fullest. Your special time might be when you take your shower or bath, when you get dressed in the morning, a meal, or perhaps sitting or walking in the garden or park. Extend and enlarge your enjoyment—really make the most of the occasion you choose.*

*For example, for a sense session in the garden or park, wear your favorite clothes, old or new. Choose your route, and as you go along, take in all the detail of the plants and flowers, their perfume, texture, growth habit, color. Notice any animals or insects and watch them intently, noticing how they move and what they are doing. Be totally involved in their activities. Smell the air, notice the wind, the sun, the clouds. Notice the surface you are on and how it feels and sounds. Perhaps have a drink or snack to indulge your sense of taste. Try to have a sense of awareness of yourself also—your feet on the surface beneath you and your breath as it flows in and out. Feel fully alive and at one with all around you.*

*Plan to have a sense session often.*

## Lighten It Up

Our sense of humor can become rusty, like any of our other senses, and thus it is obviously helpful to make time deliberately to invoke laughter. Also, if you spend your time sharpening up your funny bone, you will have less time for other emotions and will improve the general quality of your life. We can all take life too seriously, and these days experts agree that laughter is good for us. One effect of laughing is the same as that of relaxation—it encourages our bodies to produce those pain-relieving endorphins, the body's own natural painkillers. So, make a real effort to include more laughter in your life and, above all, be ready to laugh at yourself and the tangles you get yourself into.

You could make a collection of humorous books, cartoons, videos and DVDs, tapes or CDs, and so on and plan to enjoy them often. Take care over what you watch on TV; many programs, especially the news, can have a negative, depressing effect. Choose instead programs that will uplift you rather than worry you.

Humor will always lighten a tense atmosphere, so encourage it whenever you can. Sometimes when we find ourselves upset by an incident involving another person, we can change our response by altering how we think about it. Use your imagination and be quietly wicked!

*Imagine the person who has upset you being in a totally ridiculous situation. In your imagination, give him or her silly clothes to wear. Be as inventive as you like; give him a red nose, a clown's hat, or fluorescent cycling shorts. Be wild. See the person behaving in a crazy way, making a fool of himself: perhaps tripping over or climbing on a table and dancing in the middle of a meeting! Then imagine the person in the situation that upset you. This will throw a totally different light upon the situation and you will feel so much better.*

### Talk It Out

Finally, remember to *talk* about your feelings. If family or friends aren't around when you need to talk and express your feelings, use your imaginative powers.

*Imagine that in the chair opposite you is an old and trusted friend to whom you can say anything at all. Tell your friend what is on your mind and what is in your heart. Be completely frank and say it all. You may even be able to take this a stage further and visualize changing places with your friend and actually "becoming" your friend. You can physically change places, if you like, and imagine you are now that wise friend looking back at you—then give yourself advice, just as the old friend would.*

No, it's not madness to start talking to yourself in this way. Verbalizing our feelings is extremely therapeutic, as we often don't even know what it is we are really feeling until we come to put it into words. The answers to our problems are already inside us. Use this device to get in touch with, and use, your own inner truth and knowledge.

## Touch

One of the most therapeutic acts of all is for us to express our emotions positively with the physical touch of another living creature—best of all, a hug with family or friends. See if you can make a practice of either giving someone a hug every day or stroking and petting an animal. Let the person or pet know how you feel. Show your love and say thank you—just for being who she is. Remember, we *all* want and need to be loved and appreciated.

There are many techniques and ideas in this unit. Read them through or dip in and out. Try any of the ideas that particularly appeal to you. Come back to the unit again and again.

All these techniques are within your own powers to achieve. Your inner wisdom is always there to help you—let it do so.

## ACTION GUIDELINES

1. Try to become aware of when you are getting caught up in an emotional situation and use the "STOP," Magic Capsule, Cloak of Invincibility, or Grounding tactics to help stop the emotions from building up.
2. Use the Seeking Understanding Within technique to help you to cope with a problem.
3. Face and *accept* emotion that comes from your reaction to a situation.

    STOP and . . .
    *Feel the feelings.*
    *Face,* don't fight the feelings.
    *Accept* and *allow* the physical and emotional reactions.
    *Watch* and *wait,* as an observer.
    *Know* that the feelings and sensations will pass.

4. If you feel like crying, cry; if you feel angry, beat up a pillow. Alternatively, write your emotions out of your system. Try not to

vent your emotions on those close to you. Change a negative mood as quickly as you can with a positive action.

5. Keep a note of any techniques you particularly like so that when you hit a difficult patch, you have reference on how to handle it.

6. Remember that we cannot change other people—we can only change ourselves.

7. Talk your emotions through, either with family, friends, self-help groups, or a professional doctor or counselor; or try the "imaginary friend" tactic described on page 94.

8. Others cannot guess what it is you want. Tell them in a straightforward manner. Say how you feel, or express your wants and needs with an "I" statement. Begin, "I feel upset . . ." or "I would like . . ."

9. Make a list of where you obtain emotional support. Include any family, friends, doctors, counselors, self-help groups, and so on. Do you need extra support? Make a list of whom to ask for information and investigate any possibilities.

10. Consider giving *your* support to others. It is through helping others and making a contribution to life that we feel fulfilled. Can any of your skills, past or present, be useful in helping others?

11. Always foster positive emotions—by seeking, and maximizing, positive emotions, we improve our emotional life and encourage our natural healing processes to flow. Keep your sense of humor exercised.

12. Be compassionate toward yourself—always.

# UNIT 6

■

# Finding the
# Stillness Within

## CONTENTS

# Finding the
# Stillness Within

## SITTING IN STILLNESS

Sitting in Stillness is a wonderful way to bring relaxation and peace of mind into your life. It has the potential to maximize your natural healing abilities and to support you physically and emotionally. Although the technique refers to "sitting," if sitting causes you difficulties, you may, of course, lie down instead. Many people choose Sitting in Stillness, or variations of it, both for their pain management needs and as a support system for stressful times.

Just sitting, in stillness, can bring extraordinary benefits during the session itself. Its value can also spill over into everyday life and have beneficial effects upon many aspects of our whole being. Sitting in this way is very different from the relaxation method used in Unit 1. This time we are learning to stay alert, noticing what is going on, and yet still retaining a relaxed poise.

Sitting in Stillness has many benefits, including the following:

- We gain tolerance toward ourselves, others, and the situation in which we find ourselves.
- We feel more awake and alert, yet relaxed.
- We take pleasure from the smallest detail of our day.
- We learn to respond to situations and events in a calm manner.
- Our ability to concentrate improves.
- We see problems more clearly and find solutions more easily.

- We make rational decisions about what we really need to do in particular circumstances.
- All our body functions improve, including our immune system and natural healing systems.
- We find a strong center of calmness within ourselves even when our minds are in turmoil.
- We learn to approach our pain with compassion and, through our breath, soften and dissipate it.

When we learn how to sit in stillness, we can give ourselves our full attention; we do not often do this. In the middle of all our activity, we can stop for a while and regain peace and serenity, making that short space of time really count for us. We all tend to rush around during our day, putting pressure on ourselves to complete all our tasks, even if they are things we *like* doing and have chosen to do. We may often think we are running out of time during the day because we have given ourselves so much to do. Or, it is possible that, if we can't do very much physically, we put pressure on ourselves with our thoughts and feelings.

If we are lost in our thoughts and our activities, we miss many precious moments through not being fully "awake" and aware of the present. Think of the times you have done a job on automatic pilot and, at the end of it, wondered where you have "been" and what you were thinking about. Meanwhile, the world around you went by completely unnoticed. It is all too easy for us to live our lives in a sort of half-awake daze like this, living with constant repetitions of our many thoughts, which are often anxious thoughts of the future or worried thoughts about the past. By living in this way, we may miss all those tiny but wonderful events during our busy days, such as the shape of a flower, the pattern of a bird in flight, the activities of a bee, cloud formations and the color of the sky, the relaxed way a cat moves, the smell of a plant as we pass it, raindrops on a windowpane, a beautiful painting, pleasing architecture, the sound of birdsong in the silence among the noises of traffic passing, and so on. It is the recognition and the adding up of these quiet moments that can make the difference between a rushed and frantic day and a contented, satisfying day.

When we learn to become attentive to ourselves, we become more fully alive, calm, and peaceful. We become more aware of what is going on both within and outside us, accepting it as it is, without trying to change it in any way. As we continue to practice the method, we learn to lead fuller, more enjoyable lives. We develop a deep sense of ourselves and our connectedness with everything around us in our world and are content to be who we really are. We go beyond all the wants and desires of the everyday world to the true, quiet center of ourselves where there is always peace and stillness.

It sounds easy, just to sit in stillness and gain all these benefits. However, like most things worth having, we do have to learn a little about it to understand what is going on. This is because when we do sit in stillness, we become aware that our minds produce a never-ending cascade of thoughts in which it is all too easy to become entangled. This is perfectly normal: our minds *do* produce endless thoughts one after another; it's just that we don't usually notice. Sitting in stillness with nothing to do allows all these thoughts and feelings to push to the forefront of our attention. After a minute or two of just sitting, we would probably start to get fidgety and want to move or get up. So, to help us pay attention, we choose a focus for our minds. We give our minds something to hold on to, something to go back to when we become aware that our attention has wandered. This focus for our attention could be a simple design, a flower, a word or phrase, a sound, a doorknob, anything. However, as a basic practice, we are going to pay attention to the inflow and outflow of our breath. Our breath is a very convenient focus, as it is always there available to us and doesn't require any special preparations of any kind. All that is needed is a quiet, comfortable place in which to sit or lie down.

## SIT AND BREATHE

This is the basic technique for Sitting in Stillness.

*Find a quiet, comfortable place where you can be undisturbed for as long as you need (from five to fifteen or twenty minutes). You can sit or lie down, but be aware that if you lie down, you may fall asleep. To be successful with Sit and Breathe, you must be very much awake. There's no need to sit in any special way, but do sit up as straight as you can without causing any extra muscular tension. This is to help you remain alert. You can rest your head if you want to. The main thing is to be comfortable, but not so relaxed that you doze off.*

*Close your eyes and take your attention to your abdomen and notice its rise and fall as your breath enters and leaves your body.*

*Travel in your mind around your body, relaxing and letting go of each part as you come to it. Start with your feet and move up through your body, finishing with your head and face.*

*Breathing through your nose, become aware of your breath as it enters and leaves your body. Don't try to alter it in any way; just follow it as it flows in and out. Notice any movement in your chest and body, and then follow your breath as, in its own time, it flows out again through your nose. Just sit and observe it.*

*When you notice that your attention is no longer on your breath, just note the thoughts and, without criticizing yourself or getting impatient, let the thoughts go and gently bring your attention back to your breath again.*

*Continue like this, starting with a five-minute practice and building up to at least ten minutes every day, preferably fifteen to twenty. You can check the time every now and then if you want to. When the time is up, open your eyes and remain in stillness for a short while, enjoying the feelings you have generated. Take these peaceful, calm feelings with you as you slowly recommence activity.*

## Success with Sit and Breathe Practice

There's no need to worry about how you're doing: all that matters is that you're doing it. The best way to view the practice is: "I don't know if this will work, but let's see what happens." An attitude like this is one of the most important aspects of the whole exercise. It helps to stop us from being judgmental or critical and allows us to approach the practice with an open mind.

Everyone can benefit from the practice of Sitting in Stillness. You don't have to be a certain kind of person; it is an ability we are born with. Like many of our other abilities, to improve we need practice and yet more practice. As you progress, you will find your levels of attention and concentration improving and you will become generally more alert and aware of your world. If, in your practice, you bring an attitude of loving-kindness toward yourself, this will develop into a more compassionate view of others and the world. It really doesn't take very long before the benefits of this Sitting in Stillness practice overflow into your whole daily life, enhancing more and more moments of it. You may find yourself able to maintain a quiet center of calmness in the midst of all kinds of difficult episodes in your life.

### *Your Wandering Mind*

Sitting in this way is a meditation, a meditation known as mindfulness. Meditation just means paying attention, and mindfulness is as it sounds: we are paying full and total attention to the breath; our minds are full of our breath and, at times, nothing else. When you are sitting in this way, mindfully meditating on the breath, your mind *will* wander. What matters is how you deal with it when it does. What is important is the quality of *how* you bring your attention back to your focus, your breath. When you do find you have "been away," following a thought, bring your attention gently back to your breath, without criticizing yourself in any way. Just notice that your attention has wandered and focus again on the breath. Do this as many times as is necessary, without fighting or struggling with the thoughts, simply observing them, letting them go, and then going back to the breath. You may have to do this twenty, fifty, or one hundred times, it doesn't matter. The thoughts will gradually slow down and you will be able to extend your sitting time as you become more practiced. This wandering and bringing back of attention happens to everyone, no matter who she is or for how many years she has been practicing.

You may begin to realize that no matter what the thoughts are, they are just thoughts and you don't *have* to follow them. You will gradually learn to notice the thoughts as they arise and be able to let them pass without grasping at them. Meditation is not about trying to *stop* these thoughts and feelings as they come into your mind. They are not "wrong" or "bad"; our minds *do* produce thoughts one after another, it's just the way the mind works. All your different body parts have their own function. Your stomach digests your food, your lungs exchange oxygen for carbon dioxide, your heart pumps blood around your body, and your mind produces thoughts; that is its job. Your thoughts are not *you,* any more than your stomach is you.

The real you is the consciousness behind the thoughts, and you do not have to respond to the thoughts if you do not want to. You have *choice;* you can choose to follow them or you can choose to dismiss them. Your consciousness, the "You" behind your thoughts, can choose which path to take. Once you can appreciate that thoughts are not *you,* not part of you like straight or curly hair, but are produced by you, and you do not have to be at their mercy, you will have gained some most powerful knowledge.

As you meditate, you may notice that your thoughts change from one subject to another many times but certain thoughts return again and again. Note what type of thoughts these recurrent ones are—and let them go. When we are being mindful in this way, we are not trying to interfere with, censor, or suppress our thoughts. The only thing we are seeking to control is our *attention:* our attention to our breath. We are not striving to "get anywhere" or to feel in a special way. We are allowing ourselves to be just what we *are* in that moment and the next moment and the next, without interfering in any way. So, we are not trying to be calm, happy, or spiritually uplifted somehow; we are just being *as we are:* that is, fully awake and conscious, alert to this moment now. We are accepting whatever is around and in us, whether it is painful or pleasurable; we are not fighting or suppressing reality. We should not try to analyze or stop thoughts or feelings in any way, no matter what they are, but just accept them as they are and let them go. They could be about pain, memories from the past, anxieties or plans for the future, snippets of songs or conversations, the next meal, pleasurable sensations, or anything else. Thoughts and feelings pass far more quickly, no matter how strong they seem at the time, if we can accept them as they are, as just *thoughts*. Because we are not our thoughts but instead the consciousness behind the thoughts, we can *choose* whether or not we respond to them. Whatever the thoughts are, we should just continue to observe them calmly, remaining mindful of the breath.

## *A Sense of Lightness*

This directing and maintaining of attention to the breath can be very tiring, especially at first, which is why we need to start with short sessions of just a few minutes, gradually building up to longer sitting times as we continue to practice. It can also be helpful to approach the meditation with a sense of lightness. Meditation isn't meant to be a heavy, serious time. Try sitting with a relaxed mouth, with your lips barely touching in a half smile, with your tongue lying gently in the bottom of your mouth. By maintaining this expression, a message of "Be serene" will be passed to your inner being. The half smile will help you to release any tension and to feel more open, letting the session develop and flow as it will without interference from you.

## *Dealing With Discomfort*

If you find that you become aware of discomfort during the meditation, try approaching it in the following way.

> *As you breathe, be totally aware of your breath and follow it as you take the breath right into the pain. Keep your attention and your breathing right there, in and around the area of discomfort. Let your breath be your focus as you inhale and exhale. Keep your attention on your breath all the while, as it flows in and out of the pain. Continue breathing in and out of the painful area until you notice the sensations easing or changing. This may sound like a difficult task, but by confronting the discomfort in this way the area relaxes and eases. If we take the opposite path of trying to ignore or reject the pain, we tend to tighten the area, which, of course, causes us further discomfort. So, be bold. Take your breath to the pain and breathe healing warmth and relaxation into it.*

*If you really do need to move because of the intensity of the pain, don't do anything at first. Just* STOP *before you do anything; this will give you a chance to move in an organized, gentle way instead of possibly aggravating the situation by jumping about violently! Then, think what you are going to do, and move the part of the body,* intentionally, *being totally aware of what you are doing. Breathe into the part for a little while and then continue with your Sit and Breathe practice.*

## VARIATIONS OF THE BASIC METHOD

Practice Sit and Breathe every day for at least a month. When you can retain your attention on your breath fairly steadily and know you don't "disappear" with your thoughts for long periods of time, you may want to try the following variations.

### Say and Breathe

As an alternative to Sit and Breathe, you may prefer to use the following Say and Breathe meditation sometimes. It can be particularly helpful if you have a lot of discomfort. All the basic ideas are the same, but instead of using your breath as a focus for your attention, use a carefully selected word or phrase of your own choice. This can be said either out loud or silently, inside your head. It will help to stop your mind from following the thoughts as they arise in your consciousness. Use your word or phrase in conjunction with your breath as it flows in and out . . . in and out . . . in and out . . . over and over again.

> *Repeat your chosen word(s) on the out breath. Choose something really meaningful to you; it may vary from occasion to occasion, depending upon how you feel. For example:*
> *Breathe in . . . breathe out/"**Peace**". . .*

or

> *Breathe in. . . breathe out/"**I am calm.**". . .*
> *Continue with your chosen word(s) for as long as you like, anything from a few minutes to, say, twenty. As before, if*

*unwanted thoughts intrude, just let them go and come back to your words.*

### Listen and Breathe

You can extend your meditation practice to include awareness of breathing *and* another subject. This kind of practice, keeping an awareness of your breathing while also being involved with something else, is how you can incorporate the benefits of meditation and body awareness in an active way with your daily life. Try the technique at first in a fairly formal way, with a specific focus in mind; later you can try it in any situation you like. First of all, try the technique when you are listening to music, perhaps a quiet, favorite piece of your own or some music from, say, the radio. Again, the basic process is the same as for Sit and Breathe, but this time keep an awareness of your breath *and* of the music.

*Follow your breath for a few moments as in the Sit and Breathe practice and then continue by keeping an awareness of your breath and of the music, without letting the music take you over. Listen to the tone, texture, and shape of the music—and the silences between the notes. The idea is not to get lost in the music but to stay back from it sufficiently to remain mindful of your breath. If your attention wanders, when you notice it has, just gently return your focus to your breath at first and then include the music again as well. Continue to Listen and Breathe in this way for as long as you like.*

### Walk and Breathe

This is a very useful practice because it will help in ordinary movements: walking around the house or the garden, when shopping, at work, and so on. These are occasions when we tend to rush, always *going* somewhere, thinking about what we will be doing next rather than *how* we are getting there. Instead, by being aware of your body when you are walking, the walking itself becomes the aim, the focus for your attention, bringing you into the present. You will find yourself less rushed and able to move in a calm, more organized fashion. This can only be helpful to you, especially if you are hurting in any way. If there are difficulties with walking, the paying of full attention to the process will be of benefit and your walking abilities may well improve as a result. If you do have a limit on your walking distance, be sure you don't overdo it. It doesn't matter if you can walk a few steps or five miles as long as you are being mindful of your body while you practice Walk and Breathe.

When you start, it is quite a good idea to slow your pace very slightly so you can really become aware of your body's movements. After some practice at a slower pace, you can try the Walk and Breathe practice at your normal speed and at a fast rate. This will enable you to incorporate the benefits of the practice into your usual routines.

You may have never thought about the mechanics of walking before. What actually happens is that we balance first on one leg and then on the other, with our body weight poised perfectly over the foot on the ground. Quite an act!

Try the Walk and Breathe meditation as follows:

*As you walk, look ahead but be fully aware of your feet. Walk as tall as you can, but do not stiffen in any way. Some people like to imagine a golden thread going from the top of their head up into the sky, connecting with the very heart of the universe. Allow your feet, ankles, legs, hips, shoulders, and arms to stay relaxed and easy. As you walk, be aware of your feet from the heel to the toe as they peel off the ground, one after the other, step by step. Be really conscious of the contact of the ground underneath each foot and be attentive to the changing sensations from heel to toe of each foot as you walk along.*

*Once you have walked for a while with attention to your feet, you can add an awareness of your whole body, including your breath as it flows in and out. Keep the walking as relaxed as you can, especially around the hips and shoulders. Allow your arms to swing loose and free. You can also take an interest in what is around you as you move along. This is a tall order, but keep practicing and you will find a new joy in just walking as an end in itself.*

### Be and Breathe

The next technique encourages a general awareness of what is around you while you maintain attention to yourself at the same time. You can practice general awareness at any time, no matter what you are doing; washing up, brushing your teeth, eating, walking, shopping, driving, anything. It will help you to stay calm and totally in the present, fully conscious of exactly what you are doing. You will also become more aware of your body and how you are using it. By being fully aware of what you are doing, it can help you to slow down, take more care of yourself, and become less likely to aggravate any painful condition. This technique can be of great help if pain fills your whole consciousness. By concentrating upon *exactly* what you are doing, you will be able to cope with "this moment" continuously, paying attention to this moment, then the next moment, and the next, and so on. I often use this method when the pain is really intense. The following example shows how to use the technique when washing the dishes.

*Be fully aware of exactly how you are moving, of your breath and all the sensations involved in the process. Observe the water and the bubbles and watch how they behave. Notice all the colors, shapes, and sizes they make. Watch your hand reaching for the next plate. Really see the plate's color and shape, notice the glaze on the surface and any pattern on the plate. Watch the sponge or brush in your hand as you move it toward the plate and notice everything about the sponge or brush: the color, the shape, and the sensation against your hand. Be aware of your feet on the ground and the sink you are leaning over. Notice if there are any smells associated with the task. Continue to observe and to be alive to all the sensations of the whole process, maintaining as much contact with the present, with what is actually happening now, as you can.*

*At moments of great stress, some people even describe what they are doing, inside their heads or out loud. For example, "I hold the slippery plate in my left hand. It is shiny with a green- and blue-flowered pattern around the edge. My feet are firmly on the ground. My breath is slow and calm. The bubbles have tiny rainbows in them and burst as I touch them. . . ."*

As mentioned previously, you can use this type of general awareness at any time with any activity, not only if you are in discomfort. This is a way of adding great strength and pleasure to your life, of feeling deeply in touch with and part of life itself.

## MAINTAINING AWARENESS

If you are able to do so, try joining a meditation group, as it is most helpful to learn and practice with others. The meditations in this book are simply body and mind awareness techniques and have nothing to do with any kind of religion or movement. There are many groups in existence these days that are not linked with a religious movement, but some may be. The practice of some types of meditation is a very ancient and revered part of many religious movements. So do ask first, and then choose whichever type of group suits your needs.

The majority of people can't expect, or even need or want, to be able to be totally aware of their breath and body *all* the time. Often our mind is taken up by planning, analyzing, being creative, and all the other normal functions of the brain. However, even when we are busy with something else, it is helpful if we can keep an eye on our breath and body. This is rather like having an ear half-cocked for a sound if we have a baby to care for. If we can maintain this background of general awareness of ourselves, it will help us to keep in touch with our own needs and also with that center of peace and calm within us.

If you can only manage a five-minute session a day, or even one minute now and then, you will still gain from being quietly in touch with yourself. Do what you can. Go gently with yourself. By spending as much time as you can being in the present, fully conscious, you will lay a foundation of tranquillity in your life, becoming more and more in contact with your natural self and your inner wisdom as you practice finding the stillness within.

## ACTION GUIDELINES

1. Start by using the Sit and Breathe mindfulness meditation. Practice every day for as long as you can, building up from five minutes to fifteen or twenty. Do this for at least a month, longer if possible. The more strongly based your initial practice, the better the stead in which it will stand you. You will be able to cope more easily at times of real need when you remember to return to and stay with your breath.

2. Once you can keep your attention fairly steadily on your breath, try some of the other methods in this unit.

3. You may mix your meditation practice with any relaxation method so you are doing one or the other each day, or, perhaps, meditating in the morning and using a relaxation exercise in the afternoon or evening.

4. Join a group to practice meditation if you can.

5. Read books about meditation.

# UNIT 7

■

# Pacing and Planning Your Activities

## CONTENTS

# Pacing and Planning Your Activities

## MAKING A PACING PROGRAM

This unit shows you how to pace, plan, and manage your activities by building your own personal Pacing Program. Making a structured Pacing Program and setting goals for yourself are two of the most rewarding skills for you to learn. The power you gain from taking responsibility for yourself and your pain in this way gives you increased confidence and respect for yourself. This positive attitude encourages your body's natural healing processes to operate normally and effectively, allowing healing and regeneration to take place. Life will become easier for you and you will have a superb feeling of being in charge of your situation, feeling proud of yourself for coping in this way.

Most of us tend to keep going at a task until we are *forced* by the pain to stop. A Pacing Program will ensure that you stop *before* the pain arises. By pacing yourself and learning how to set carefully planned goals, you will be able gradually to achieve more and increase your activities in a structured way . . . *without increasing the pain level.* Pacing will save you from seesawing between doing too much, then, as a result, being able to do hardly anything. When we throw ourselves from one end of the seesaw to the other in this all-or-nothing way, we find we aren't in control of our pain and that it is controlling us. Having a Pacing Program means you can increase your activity but at the same time keep pain levels under control. Some of the things you want to do may take longer but you will be doing what you aim to do success-fully, without stirring up pain. You are going to find a balanced way between too much rest and too much action. Through carefully devised and structured goals, you will also be able to make progress with your physical activities. This is an ideal way, for example, to increase your walking or sitting abilities, if that is your need.

If you can, it is good to involve your family and friends with your program. Tell them you are starting a new program to reduce your pain levels and they are not to be surprised if you stop doing a job in the middle and leave it until later. If you tell them everything is under con-trol and things will get done but in a different way from before, they will understand. They will be delighted to hear you are taking an active part in caring for yourself and even more pleased when they start to see results. Soon they will see improvements not only in your well-being but also in your involvement in a wider range of activities. If it isn't appropriate to involve anyone else, you can work perfectly well at your program independently.

It will take a week or so of fairly intensive detective work to find out all you can about how your pain relates to your activities. You will then be able to make up a program to work from. Once you have done this, you will only need to spend a few minutes once a week just to review how you are doing and to set your goals for the next week.

The content of your Pacing Program will depend upon your own physical requirements and your own personal situation. Many people may not need to make major adjustments to their life, perhaps only to be more aware of planning ahead more carefully and changing activi-ties fairly regularly during the day. However, some people may need to make quite a few changes over a period of a few weeks or months. You will have to be your own judge about this, as only you know your own circumstances.

The whole program is very full and comprehensive and there are many activities for you to do. Remember, all the way through the pro-gram, to do just *one step at a time*. Concentrate on the step you are working with and the rest of the program will fall into place in its own time. There is no hurry and you can complete the program as is convenient for you. Keep going, as the end result will be success with one of the most worthwhile skills you have ever learned.

## STEP 1: A POSITIVE RELATIONSHIP WITH THE PAIN

The key to natural pain relief is to forge a positive relationship with your body and the part that hurts: not fighting it, hating it, or regarding it as an enemy, but nurturing a compassionate, befriending relationship in which you learn how to take care of your pain's needs. The more closely attuned you become to your body, the more you will be able to work with it in aiming for the reduction of pain. The part of you that is hurting needs your positive, constructive attention in the form of care, consideration, and empathy.

Your body, once you tune in to the right wavelengths, speaks to you and can tell you in its own way what it needs and wants. This is often manifested in physical sensations of one kind or another. When your body is working happily, it lets you know by giving you positive sensations: those of being relaxed, bright, at ease when moving and with a glowing sensation of good health. When you have pain, your body is telling you it is unhappy, and that it wants you to treat the part that is hurting with respect. The first step is to become more aware of your body, using the following technique to develop a positive relationship with the part that is in pain. You will be rewarded by a deeper knowledge and understanding of yourself and be in a better position to control and reduce the pain in the next stages of the Pacing Program.

### The Stop and Change Technique

*When you become aware of the pain and realize your body is trying to gain your attention,* STOP. *Immediately* STOP *what you are doing and take note of what your body is trying to let you know. It is clamoring for your attention in the only way it knows. You may find it useful to actually say, either out loud or inside your head,* "STOP."

*Having made this space for yourself by stopping what you are doing, take your attention to your breathing and let it become a little slower and deeper for a few moments. Then build a relationship with the part that hurts; talk, inside your head, or even out loud if you prefer, directly to the part in a kindly way, just as you would talk to a small child needing comfort.*

*For example: "Thank you for letting me know you're not up to doing anymore right now. I'll stop for a while and give you a rest. We can do some more later. Now, let's see if we can make you more comfortable."*

*If you'd like, make physical contact with the part needing special attention. If it is convenient and comfortable to do so, put a hand over the special place; this will tell the area that you are wanting to communicate with it.*

*Now become aware of your breath again and spend a few moments just watching it as it flows in and out; feel warmth and relaxation begin to spread around your whole body.*

*And then, on each in breath, imagine your breath going straight to the part needing attention, taking warmth and relaxation with it. Continue to breathe this warmth and relaxation into this area for a while. This will calm and reduce the pain.*

*And now that you have gained, literally, "a breathing space,"* CHANGE *your activity. Change to a different one, one giving the affected part some respite.*

This is the beginning of a relationship with the special area of your body and with the pain—a partnership or friendship even. With the later steps in the Pacing Program, you will discover how to stop and change activities *before* the pain increases—this is the true art of pacing.

### The Pressure of Time

Many of us feel the pressure of time upon us. We may feel we have too much to do in the time available or, when we are involved in a job, we have "got" to finish it. On the other hand, some of us who have to rest our bodies may feel as though we have too much time. Time can, therefore, be a pressure upon us for different reasons. For those of us who find we have too much time, we can take the opportunity of the extra time given to us, in meditating, with visualizations, or with any of the other wonderful ways in which we can develop our inner strengths and powers. We can still enjoy our lives and make the most of every moment, being appreciative of what we *do* have and *can* do, whatever our situation. When we are involved and enjoying ourselves, time seems to speed up and pass faster, because time is relative to what we are doing. When we meditate, time appears to cease to exist altogether and each and every moment becomes timeless.

When we are pushed for time to complete a task, or feel we really have to press on with a task, we will serve ourselves, and the task, better if we are firm about stopping and changing activities when our body tells us to. If you find that you have a tendency to continue with the task even after receiving strong messages from your body, ask yourself the questions below. When asking the questions, relax and allow your natural inner wisdom to surface, accepting the very first thoughts, ideas, or pictures that come to you. The answers appearing in your mind will allow you to see the whole picture and so put everything in perspective. You will discover that usually it doesn't actually matter if you do stop for a moment, and the "worst" is nothing very terrible after all.

*"What would happen if I stopped now?"*
Next ask, *"Does it really matter?"*
Last ask, *"What is the worst that could happen?"*

When you are feeling the pressure of deadlines or urgency in this way, it will help if you can come into the moment, the "now": being fully aware of the present, not the future of the deadline. By becoming aware of the process itself, the doing of the task, you take the pressure from yourself. When we concentrate on doing the best we can, at this very moment, pain considerations included, we forget about deadlines.

You can say to yourself,

*"Life is not an emergency."*
And then, *"There is plenty of time."*
Or even, *"I enjoy this minute because I'm in it."*

These affirmations, when repeated with real conviction, will help to change the way you think, supporting and nourishing your inner being.

## STEP 2: KEEPING A DIARY

The second step of the Pacing Program is to spend about a week keeping a diary of your activities. The diary can take the form of a list of very rough notes or jottings. There is no need to write a lengthy entry each day, unless that is your desire. You do need to keep the diary regularly, with entries every day for this period, noting down everything you do during the day. This diary is going to give you much information about how you currently organize your days. It is best if you give as much detail as possible because, obviously, the more information you put into the diary, the more useful the information you will be able to glean from it. With this information you will be in a strong position to make some judgments about how exactly you spend your time.

### *How to Fill the Diary*

You will need a personal notebook, exercise book, or loose-leaf file for your diary and for the records you will make during the Pacing Program.

> *For about a week, make a note of everything you do, as you do it; include mealtimes, mundane tasks, watching TV, traveling time, rest periods, and so on. Record how long you spend on each activity, especially any rest periods. Also note any highs and lows of emotional feelings.*
>
> *Remember—every time you change your activity, write it down. It's quite a commitment but it's only for a week and it is a vital first step in your program. At the end of each day, mark your activities as follows:*
>
> - *Mark any activity that made you feel better in any way whatsoever, especially if it helped to reduce your pain levels, with a star. You don't need to star the rest periods because we aim gradually to reduce these as far as possible over the coming weeks.*
> - *Mark any activity where your body made itself heard with additional pain, either during or after the activity, with a small circle.*
> - *Mark any activity that you completed reasonably easily*

*and which caused no real change to "normal" pain levels with a check.*

- *Mark all rest periods with R.*

At the end of a week or so, you will have gained much information about your current activity pattern. You will now be able to use your notes to make valuable discoveries to help you to pace and plan your activities.

### A Sample Diary

An extract from the diary of a friend of mine, Lucy, is given on page 120. Remember, this is an example only; your diary will look completely different. This extract is to show you how the layout may look.

## STEP 3: SORTING OUT ACTIVITIES

Once you have collected some details about how you spend your time, you can start to examine the information for ways in which you can consider making some changes.

*First of all, draw up a chart with headings similar to the one on page 121 to find out if there is a pattern to your activities. Categorize your activities in lists under each of the headings.*

- *One list for the activities that caused extra pain, those marked with a circle.*
- *Another list for those activities marked with a check; these were the "safe" activities causing no real change in pain levels.*

Looking at the diary extract, we can see that Lucy overdid things when she went for a long shopping expedition followed by going visiting later in the day. She then had to rest for most of the remainder of the day.

- *A third list will be of those activities marked with a star, where you gained benefit by feeling better.*
- *Finally, make a separate note of rest periods each day.*

The example on page 121 was taken from the list compiled from Lucy's diary. Again, her list will be completely different from yours. It is only an example of the way to extract and categorize information from the diary of activities.

# STEP 4: DETECTIVE WORK

Find a quiet time of day when you won't be disturbed and arrange to make yourself as comfortable as possible; it is time for some detective work on your lists.

When Lucy investigated her lists, she noticed that the activities where she felt her body needed more support fell into fairly simple categories. These were activities that involved sitting, bending, and walking for any

## EXTRACT FROM LUCY'S DIARY

| Date: August 5 | Time Taken | Check/Circle/Star/R |
|---|---|---|
| 7:30 a.m., woke, washed, and dressed | 20 | √ |
| Made breakfast | 15 | ☆ |
| Breakfast | 15 | ☆ |
| Got ready to go out and tidied house | 45 | √ |
| Drove car (excited) | 15 | O |
| Shopping | 90 | O |
| Drove car | 15 | O |
| Rest | 60 | R |
| Lunch | 45 | √ |
| Rest | 30 | R |
| Went visiting | 90 | O |
| Rest | 60 | R |
| Potted plants (felt contented) | 20 | ☆ |
| Rest | 60 | R |
| Prepared dinner | 30 | √ |
| Dinner | 30 | √ |
| Cleaned kitchen | 30 | √ |
| Ironing (tired and depressed) | 40 | O |
| Whole evening spent lying down | 180 | R |
| Went to bed about 10:30 p.m. | | |

## EXTRACT FROM LUCY'S LISTS

| Circle (extra pain) | Check (no great change from "normal" pain) | Star (reduced pain) |
|---|---|---|
| Bending in garden (15 mins. weeding) | Washing/dressing | Entertained friends at my house |
| Driving car, 15 mins. | Short bus ride | Relaxation session |
| Concert, 2 hrs. | Watching TV | Walked ¼ mile |
| Walked ½ mile | Preparing meals | Potting plants |
| Shopping, 1½hrs. | Eating meals | TV comedy show |
| Visited friends (uncomfortable chair) | | Fed ducks |
| Argument with son over untidy room | | Watched children playing |

## REST PERIODS

| Date | Length (minutes/hours) | Total Number | Total Time |
|---|---|---|---|
| August 3 | 60, 30, 60, 60, 60, 3½ hrs. | 6 | 8 hrs. |
| August 4 | 30, 10, 15, 60, 20, 10, 2 hrs. | 7 | 4 hrs. 25 mins. |

distance. She decided she spent too long on many of her activities. For instance, she felt the shopping expedition was too strenuous for her and would be better split into two outings. She noticed that she could regularly walk for a quarter of a mile with ease but not much farther without additional pain. Lucy also discovered that her activities occurred in rather an erratic way. For example, one day she might go both visiting and shopping, or she might suddenly decide to walk a very long distance and then, in the next few days, not walk very far at all.

### Analyzing Your Activities

You can analyze your own activities in a similar way, finding out as much as you can about the pattern of your activities.

### Danger List

- *Look carefully at your lists marked with a circle (extra pain).*
- *What kind of activity aggravates the pain?*
- *Are the activities concerned involved with particular physical movements? (for example, bending, reaching, pushing, carrying, walking, sitting, climbing stairs)*
- *Is the length of time you spend on an activity relevant? Could you manage a shorter spell at the same activity more comfortably?*

ACTION: Take notice of what your body is telling you and adjust your movements and tasks accordingly.

### Safe List

- *Now look at the checked list of activities, those that, with care, are reasonably safe for you.*
- *Is the type of movement you use different or the same as on the other lists?*
- *Is the time spent on the activity the same or different from the other lists?*
- *What is it about these activities that makes them more comfortable for you?*

ACTION: Take notice of what your body is telling you and adjust your movements and tasks accordingly.

### Starred List

- *Look at the starred list.*
- *When your body was happy and things improved a little, what were you doing?*
- *Were all the activities "resting" activities?*
- *If the activities involved movement, what kind of movements of your body?*
- *Were the activities all of short duration?*

ACTION: Consider if it would help if you did more of these activities.

## Spacing of Activities

- *Examine your record for spacing of activities.*
- *Look at your activities overall. Did you find your commitments to be too close together during the week, perhaps on, say, a few consecutive days and then no commitments for the rest of the period?*
- *Do you tend to cram too much into one day and then do hardly anything the following day?*
- *Look at your activities during each day. Were all your main activities clustered in one part of the day?*
- *Were there activities clustered in which you used similar physical movements—for example, sitting to travel and then sitting to type and then sitting to talk to people?*
- *Do you think you carry on with individual activities for too long?*

ACTION: Rearrange your commitments to suit your body's needs.

## The Variability of Pain Levels

- *Does the pain change in any way throughout the day?*
- *Is the pain regularly fairly high in the morning and then does it ease off as you start moving around?*
- *Does the pain level build up during the day?*
- *Is the pain particularly noticeable after certain activities?*

ACTION: Organize your activities to cope with these patterns of pain.

## Emotions

- *Does the way you feel have any effect on your pain levels?*
- *Do pain levels drop when you are enjoying yourself?*
- *Do they rise when you are upset in some way?*

ACTION: Investigate new ways of handling the situations that cause you distress. Investigate how to handle your own feelings. (See Unit 5, Dealing With Your Feelings, and Unit 8, Enjoying Yourself.)

## Rest Periods

- *Are your rest periods very frequent?*
- *Do they vary in duration?*

- *Does anything rule how long they last?*
- *What do you do during a rest period?*
- *Look at which activities were followed by a rest period. Is there a pattern here?*
- *Do you tend to overdo things and then have to spend extra time resting as a consequence?*

ACTION: Consider replacing some of your rest periods with relaxation sessions or exercises. Always keep as active and mobile as possible.

See what you can discover from the pattern of your activities; now is an excellent opportunity to find out where you could consider making some really valuable changes in your life. Pacing and planning your activities will give you a tremendous and positive input to your well-being. When we talk about Pacing and Planning, we really mean managing our activities with a good balance between movement and rest—a balance also among the *types* of physical movements and activities in which we are involved. To obtain a balance may involve having to take many short breaks from what you are doing and also frequently to change the type of physical movement and activity in which you are involved—in other words, to Stop and Change your activities. The next step of the program will help you to stop and change in a very effective way, *before* the pain level rises.

Once you are aware of your activity pattern during the day and understand why you need to pace your activities, it becomes easier to start being more considerate toward your body and fulfilling its needs.

## STEP 5: TIMING YOUR ACTIVITIES

You now know that the best way to handle any painful sensations is not to struggle on with the activity in which you are involved but to Stop and Change to an activity that will give your body some respite. Even better—and this is the essence of a good Pacing Program—is to Stop and Change *before* the onset of extra pain. Stopping an activity while you are still as comfortable as when you started means that *you* are actually in control of the situation.

From now on, you are not going to wait for the uncomfortable sensations to tell you to stop what you are doing: you are going to learn how to judge when to stop an activity *before* your body tells you in a dramatic way that it needs your attention. I know this situation is unavoidable on occasions, but gradually you will have fewer and fewer of those "emergency" occasions as your Pacing Program becomes established.

Often we are not sure how long we can carry on with an activity before we need to stop. The tendency, as mentioned previously, is to continue with what we are doing until we *have* to stop. The most successful way to decide the optimum period to continue with an activity is to time it. In order to time what they are doing, most people find a countdown type of timer with a buzzer to be more effective than a watch or clock. If we rely on looking at a clock or watch, it is all too easy to become so engrossed in what we are doing that we forget all about the time.

*Take a few moments to write down the main activities where, after a short while, you are conscious of increased pain: that is, your body is giving you messages telling you it needs some respite and support. There's no need to make it a very long list; try to keep to the most important activities, such as walking, sitting, and standing. For example, Lucy made a list that included walking and driving.*

Our lists will all be different, depending upon our own individual situation. Your list may contain only one or two activities or it may include others—for example, housework, standing, sport, traveling, hobbies.

## STEP 6: FINDING YOUR BASELINE TIMES

You will have to decide for yourself how long it is reasonable to carry out the activities on your list, stopping *before* your body starts to tell you it needs to rest or change.

*Base the time on how long you can do the activity without causing yourself any more pain either during or after the activity. Be aware that pain levels can increase a few hours or even a day later because of too much activity. Be generous and begin at a much lower level than you think is right for you; in this way, you will be successful from the start. A simple method to ensure that you don't stay too long with one activity is to set a countdown timer and obey it. It may be useful to make a note of, for example, your sitting times over a few days and then choose the lowest as your baseline, even if it is only a few minutes. When finding the baseline for walking a short distance, it may be more useful to count the steps taken, instead of trying to time the walking.*

*You may also need to work out how many times a day you can safely accomplish working at this level. For instance, if you can walk, say, half a mile, you may be able to achieve it once, twice, three, or even more times a day, but you do need to know. The same applies to any other activity.*

*For example, Lucy worked out her baseline levels for walking as a quarter of a mile, twice a day, and for driving as five minutes, twice a day.*

## STEP 7: TESTING YOUR BASELINE LEVELS

Now that you have your baselines, you are all set to test them out.

*Over the next few days, stay at your baseline levels for your chosen activities. You may find this to be easier if you use a countdown timer, as mentioned before.*

*Try not to go over your baseline times; keep to them as far as you possibly can. It may even be wise to keep a little in reserve for unexpected events.*

*It is good, too, to be flexible in your pacing, as pain does vary from day to day, often for no reason you can discern. So if you are still feeling rather uncomfortable after a few days, do not hesitate to reassess your level of activity and drop down until you reach a level at which you can operate more easily.*

*It may be that you think your ultimate baseline level is very low, but don't let it concern you. The main objective at the moment is to keep pain down to a reasonable and more manageable level for a period of time. Later on you are going to build upon the level.*

Once you are satisfied with your baseline level for each of your activities, and you know how many times you can perform each activity during a day, you will be far more confident with your body. Confidence grows when you know you have found a level at which you can generally be comfortable, both during and after the activity.

## STEP 8: GETTING PAIN LEVELS UNDER CONTROL

*You can begin by making a plan for the week ahead and do this for every week until you are sure you have your pain under control. In making the plan for the week ahead, you need to take into account the ideas from this unit about finding out, and working at, a baseline level with activities; spacing out your commitments and activities; and leaving time for relaxation, exercises, enjoyment, and quietude each day.*

It is a good idea to continue with keeping a brief diary of overall activities because then you can assess your progress more easily. Also, it is an excellent idea to keep a brief record of the activities for which you have made baseline times. It will help you to keep to the times and to check your progress. The chart below is an example of Lucy's walking baseline record.

### BASELINE WALKING RECORD

**Baseline Level:** *quarter mile (about 600 steps), twice a day*

| Date | Level Achieved | Notes |
|------|----------------|-------|
| *August 15* | *600, 600* | *OK* |
| *August 16* | *600, 600* | *OK* |
| *August 17* | *600, 700* | *Pain. Too much.* |
| *August 18* | *600, 600* | *OK* |

**Comments at end of week:** *I managed to keep to my baseline quite well, apart from one day. I will give it another week before moving on to Goal Setting*

After another week, Lucy decided that her baseline level was correct for her. She also made similar records for her driving and gardening activities.

It is important to keep to your plans as far as possible. The aim is for *you* to decide what you do, not the pain. The art of pacing is to stop while you are still comfortable, and not when your body tells you to.

If, despite your pacing efforts, you have a day when your body needs some time to recover, you can still try to keep to your plans, but give yourself more rest and relaxation breaks. On the other hand, when you have a day when your body feels happy and free, you need to respect this also and not overdo things by attempting more than you planned.

At the end of each week, it is a good idea to assess the previous week and see how you fared. You can then make adjustments for the next week. Also, you deserve to praise and acknowledge your achievements, especially at the end of each successful week. Through your own efforts you are managing to keep your body on a more even keel. A small treat or reward built into the program at the successful achievement of each stage is an excellent idea as an incentive and for reinforcing your determination to make, and stick to, a pacing schedule. It doesn't matter what it is, provided it is something meaningful to *you*. It could be anything from a special visit to something more simple, like treating yourself to a favorite magazine.

Always remember that if you do deviate from your Pacing Program, it's not the end of the world. We all do what we can to the best of our ability. If you don't get it right all the time (and who could), never mind. Continue to be kind to yourself and just start again as soon as you can. Nothing will be lost; every day is a new beginning. It may help to make a note of the circumstances that caused you to deviate from your program: for example, unexpected visitors, a longer journey than expected, or just a foolhardy moment! At the end of a week or two, if you keep breaking your baseline times, you can see if there is a pattern involved. You can then ask yourself why it keeps happening and if there is anything you can do about it.

### Organizing Your Day

Some of us may feel as though there is not enough time in each day for everything we either need or want to do, whether it is work or leisure. If this is a concern, it will help us if we look at all our activities and consider reorganizing our time. We may even look at dropping certain things that are not so important in order to do what we really want to do and the things we have to do. For example, we may find that we truly don't have time to fit in something special we would like to do. If this is so, we could look at how we fill our time during the day to see if there is anything we could put aside for the moment. For instance, perhaps we could save some time by limiting our time spent watching TV or reading newspapers or magazines.

## Priority Cards

Using Priority Cards is an excellent way of enabling us to feel on top of all the many things we may have, or want, to do. By using the cards to prioritize jobs in order of their importance, we can quickly find out which activities need immediate attention and which can be left for a while.

- *Make a list of everything you consider you need and want to do in, say, the next week.*
- *Now write each of these items on a separate reminder card.*
- *Each day take time first thing in the morning to shuffle your cards into the order of importance for that day. You will be able to see at a glance which items to do that day and which can be left for another day, and also which tasks to tackle first and which may be fitted in toward the end of the day.*

Prioritizing activities like this gives us a tremendous sense of being on top of things and can help to stop feelings of pressure building.

## Saying No

Occasionally we may be asked to do something when we are too busy to fit it in, or perhaps when we are in need of some space for a period of quietness and relaxation. Saying no may come hard to us at first, especially when we say it to people we care about. It is best if we say it simply, in a straightforward manner: "No, I'm sorry, I will have to leave that for another time." There's no need to offer lots of explanations or apologies. People may be surprised when we first say no to them but they will respect us for having said what we really feel. We will also find that our answer will be accepted at face value. In fact, once we become accustomed to what, perhaps, may be a new idea for us, we may be surprised at just how easy it is to say a simple no, firmly but kindly.

Sometimes we may have to decline to take part in an activity that is really tempting to us but is outside our current abilities. This is where we need to be extra conscious of our body's requirements. It gives us another opportunity to practice a Stop and Change technique. Using the technique to say STOP or No to ourselves at these times also gives us more power and confidence, and fosters a positive attitude toward our body. We may be able to reach a compromise solution after we have said no to the activity, perhaps partaking in some aspect of the activity or planning to take it up later.

We may all, from time to time, out of frustration or anger at our situation, say to ourselves, "But I *want* to do it" or "I've *got* to do it." These thoughts are not helpful to us and it's best if we let them go; although, of course, we're only human and we all give in to this sort of desire from time to time. Another way to deal with this type of thought is to ask ourselves:

> *"Am I helping myself by doing this?"*
> *"What would happen if I didn't do this?"*
> *"Does it really matter?"*
> *"What is the worst that could happen if I didn't do this?"*

In these circumstances, the best tactic for emotional peace and for support of our physical needs is to *change* our focus to concentrate upon something we *can do*. When we do this, we can congratulate ourselves on our constructive and supportive attitude toward our body and mind, an attitude that can transform our view of ourselves and enhance our self-worth.

Learning to organize our time, make priorities, and say the occasional no are all essential aspects of a Pacing Program. These skills give us a sense of pride and purpose with an increasing feeling of control in our life, especially with the commitments we have to honor and the pastimes we choose—and, of course, over our pain levels.

Once you have things more under control, you can then move to the next exciting step, which is working toward improvement by gradually increasing the amount you do or the time you spend on each activity. However, before you go on to Goal Setting for Improvement, this is a good point to say a few words about using and moving your body.

## Using and Moving Your Body

When we have been in pain for a while, our body needs an extra physical input in order to return to being as fully fit and active as we are able to be. There may be a reluctance to start extra movement, but with careful pacing and goal setting, we can increase exercise and mobility steadily, without added pain. Exercise makes us feel better about ourselves, increases our overall mobility, and helps to reduce pain. Movement and exercise do not necessarily mean formal exercises; enjoyable and informal activities like walking, dancing, and swimming are exercise.

With this in mind, why not try moving to music, an activity that most people enjoy? This is one of the best ways to keep active, whether lying down, sitting, or on your feet. Choose slow, relaxing music and allow it to direct your movements. Remember to make this and any other exercise part of your Pacing Program, and space out your exercise throughout the day. With good pacing and goal setting, we can increase our exercise and mobility steadily, becoming as fit as we are able to be.

You may need specific exercises for your own condition and these must always be done with the supervision of an expert, such as a chiropractor, osteopath, sports trainer, or physiotherapist. Although there are many exercise books available, please be *very cautious*. In fact, it's best not to use them at all without getting professional advice first. When you have a painful condition, you need to take great care to do any exercises correctly, and this needs supervision. Exercises also need to be checked as being safe for your particular condition. Make sure any exercises you do undertake are done in a calm, meditation-like state, with awareness of how the movements affect your body. Be sensitive to the messages from your body and pay great attention to the quality of each movement. If you notice any increase in pain at any time, especially a sharp pain, stop what you are doing immediately.

You may want to consider investigating the Alexander Technique.

With a course of lessons in the technique, you will learn to move with poise and economy of movement, which will naturally help to minimize pain and strain. The Alexander Technique offers a practical approach to the way in which we move and use our body; our whole being becomes calmer as we regain the grace and ease of movement lost since childhood.

## STEP 9: GOAL SETTING FOR IMPROVEMENT

Having a successful Pacing Program means we do not always have to give up favorite, or essential, activities completely. It is often possible for us to restart old activities or begin new ones with a careful and thoughtfully organized plan. Setting goals for ourselves gives an immediate positive injection into our lives and helps us to make improvements in our activity levels in a steady and safe way. Having goals and working toward them gives us hope and confidence and boosts our self-esteem.

Having found your baseline levels for some of your activities, you can use your knowledge to move on to Goal Setting. You achieve your goal by working toward it in a succession of small steps, slowly increasing the chosen activity by a small amount in each step. This may be only by a few minutes, or a pace at a time, if walking. Please don't be over-ambitious: you want to set yourself up for success at every stage.

Each small step is called a mini-goal, which you set each week. This is a goal within the main goal. At the end of the week, you assess the previous week and set another mini-goal for the following week. By starting at a low level and making only a small increase each week, mini-goals are very achievable. You enjoy continuous success by achieving these mini-goals and thereby make sure and steady progress toward your main goal without any "hiccups." Success will become a habit. Your main goal may be broken down into as many mini-goals as you decide are necessary.

### Suggestions for Successful Goal Setting

*Select just one of your activities to work on at first. If you attempt more than one, you will not be able to monitor your progress clearly. If you are starting from a fairly inactive level, choose something relatively simple to start with. You might find it helpful to choose, say, the goal of achieving a relaxation session every day, or doing your exercises regularly. As you become stronger, more active, and more capable, you can return to other activities and set goals for them. Lucy, for example, decided to concentrate upon improving her general sitting rather than her driving, which is a more complex activity.*

*Your goals may be anything at all but choose an activity you really want to work on, and then your desire to achieve will help you to keep going toward your goal.*

*You need to set yourself very precise goals. For example, "I'll go for a walk every day" is not as effective as "I will walk down the road to the shop every day."*

*It is important to have a time element in your goals. For instance, "I will walk down the road to the shop in four weeks' time."*

*Make your goals achievable. For example, "I will drive the three hundred miles to visit my sister" is obviously far more difficult for someone who can hardly sit to drive at all at the moment than "I will drive the five miles to town and back by the end of the month."*

## STEP 10: MAKING A GOAL SHEET

Every week you will need a goal sheet similar to the one on page 134. You could photocopy this blank goal sheet if it is convenient for you; otherwise copy it into your notebook or file.

Aim for slow and steady increases toward your goal each week. Start at your baseline level of activity and add on a little extra for your first week's mini-goal. You will have to decide how much, as you know your capabilities. *Keep your mini-goals realistic;* if goals and expectations are too high, you will not be helping yourself. There is a space on the chart for a small reward each week; this may seem unimportant, but its power is not to be underestimated. Including a reward or a treat system into the weekly goal regimen really does help to motivate you and make you feel good about achieving your goal. Use it and see for yourself. The system reinforces the success at a deep level. Arrange to have a bigger reward for when you achieve your main goal. This will give you something to aim for and will acknowledge your successful completion of the main goal.

Tell your family and friends what you are doing and involve them in the project, and let them read this program if possible. Look at your diary for the best time of day for you to do physical activities and exercises. Choose times when your body is feeling most comfortable. Decide upon your first goal and write it in a notebook, as shown on the facing page.

---

### SAMPLE GOAL SHEET

MAIN GOAL:

My reward for achieving my main goal will be:

MINI-GOAL for the week:

My reward for achieving my mini-goal will be:

| Day | Daily goal | What I actually achieved | Notes |
| --- | --- | --- | --- |
| Mon | | | |
| Tues | | | |
| Wed | | | |
| Thurs | | | |
| Fri | | | |
| Sat | | | |
| Sun | | | |

How did I do this week?

Do I get my reward?

Mini-goal for next week:

## LUCY'S GOAL SHEET

**MAIN GOAL:** *To walk to the shop at the end of the road and back in six weeks' time (a little over half a mile) without extra pain.*

**My reward for achieving my main goal will be:** *A special evening out.*

**MINI-GOAL for the week:** *To walk halfway and back (about 700 steps in all).*

**My reward for achieving my mini-goal will be:** *A bag of mixed fruit and nuts and my favorite magazine.*

| Day | Daily goal | What I actually achieved | Notes |
|---|---|---|---|
| Mon | *650 steps* | *625* | *Too far, cut back* |
| Tues | *600* | *600* | *Fine. Same on Wed.* |
| Wed | *600* | *600* | *OK* |
| Thurs | *625* | *625* | *Well done* |
| Fri | *650* | *650* | *Well done* |
| Sat | *675* | *680* | *Excellent* |
| Sun | *700* | *700* | *Did it!* |

**How did I do this week?** *Very well, I stuck to my plan.*

**Do I get my reward?** *Yes!*

**Mini-goal for next week:** *To walk another 100 extra steps—800 steps in all.*

### How to Complete the Goal Sheet

At the start of the week, fill in the main goal. This will help you to keep your focus strong.

Then complete the mini-goal section. For your first week, add on a small increase to your baseline starting point for the activity. Remember, take small steps, not giant strides. You will have to decide what is reasonable for you.

Remember to complete the reward sections. It is important to celebrate your successes, acknowledging and praising your *achievements. Also, share your aims and your successes with others if you can.*

*Each day, make a brief comment in the Notes section on how you performed and then decide your next day's goal. This may be the same, lower, or slightly higher, depending upon how you coped with the current day. If you do aim slightly higher, make sure it is a small step only. Your progress path may be slightly up and down but your overall aim should be to gradually improve during the week.*

It is helpful to fill in your goal sheet every day until you successfully achieve your goal.

Lucy's first completed goal sheet looked like the one shown on page 135.

## STEP 11: ASSESSING YOUR PROGRESS

At the end of each week, assess it and ask yourself if you achieved your goal comfortably or if it was rather a struggle. Did you receive your reward or not? If your week went well, continue with your program by adding on just a small increase for the next week's mini-goal. However, if you did not achieve your mini-goal in a consistent way, you can drop back the following week to a slightly lower level, giving yourself smaller steps to take forward. Sometimes you may even need to revise the whole situation and consider whether your overall goal is too high for you. Think creatively to see if there is a way around this, perhaps slightly changing your aims for the moment.

It is rare to progress in a straight line to your goal. Sometimes progress levels off and you may reach a plateau. If this happens to you, keep your morale high by looking back through your notebook to see how you have progressed. Looking back this way ensures that you acknowledge your achievement so far; it makes you feel good and gives you confidence to go on again. At those times when you do level out, be resolute and keep on pacing yourself at that same level for a while, knowing you will be able to push forward again when your body has settled at the new level more happily. Patience, determination, and perseverance are the watchwords for successful "pacers." Meanwhile, as always, keep your spirits high by concentrating your attention on what you *can* do and by holding a strong visual image of your goal in your mind.

## STEP 12: VISUALIZING YOUR GOAL

One of the most exciting and vitally important ways in which you can help yourself to achieve your goals is to use your imagination to visualize yourself successfully accomplishing your aims. You can easily do this in the following way.

*Take a short break at a time when you can arrange to be undisturbed, and make yourself really comfortable, either sitting or lying down. Begin by closing your eyes and taking your attention to your breath. Just allow it to become a little slower and deeper. Feel the waves of relaxation begin to move through your body. Travel in your mind around your body, allowing each part in turn to become warmer, heavier, and more and more relaxed.*

*When you are fully relaxed, use your imagination to see yourself as you will be at the time when your goal is achieved. The day is perfect and everything is just right for you. You feel strong and confident, full of satisfaction and pride, knowing you have achieved your chosen goal by your own efforts. Whatever your goal is, see yourself carrying it out with ease and confidence. If it is walking, see yourself walking tall and freely. If it is sitting comfortably, see yourself sitting in a poised and relaxed position, happily engaged in some activity of your choice. Visualize yourself in your chosen activity. Have a sense of what is going on around you, what you are wearing, any colors, sounds, smells, and textures around you. If you are sitting writing, feel the pen and paper, the table, the chair; see the pen move across the paper. If you are driving, see the environment around you, see the colors and hear the sounds. Visualize and sense as much as you can about the whole scene, whatever it is. See yourself with a happy smile and know you can be this way more and more often. Feel proud of yourself for accomplishing*

*your goal and know you can go on with confidence to achieve
even greater success and fulfillment in any area you want.*

*Continue with your visualization for as long as you wish
and then slowly come back to the room, knowing you can successfully achieve this and any other goal of your choice.*

Use your visualization every day to bring your goal nearer to you. When
we see our success in our mind or sense it in our body, our goal is even
more sure to become our reality, for "What we can conceive and believe,
we can achieve."

## CONGRATULATIONS

Many, many things you had thought out of your reach can be achieved
by careful pacing, planning, and goal setting. With your new skills and
your pain in more control, you can have a superb feeling of "I did it by
myself!" The success is yours and yours alone. You deserve to succeed
and you will succeed.

At every stage during your Pacing Program, acknowledge and congratulate yourself for your achievements. Do not underestimate the
reward system built into the Goal Setting technique; it is a vital part of
the whole program. We all respond to praise—and who better to give
it to you than yourself? You are making great steps forward in gaining
control over your pain and this is an achievement that cannot be under-
rated in any way. You can be proud of yourself.

Making and keeping to a Pacing and Goal Setting Program is of vital
importance in learning how to manage pain. Bear in mind that what
you are doing is for *yourself* and will help to reduce your pain; this will
enable you to keep to your plans. Be supportive toward yourself, noncritical and nonjudgmental.

This is a wonderful opportunity to move forward—do take it.

## ACTION GUIDELINES

1. Keep in touch with your body and its needs. Use the Stop and Change technique to "talk" to your body.

2. Work through the Pacing Program. Keep to your plans so as not to overdo things when you are feeling better. Remember to concentrate on one stage at a time.

3. Set yourself a simple goal and start working toward it. Use the Goal Setting technique for an enjoyment activity as well as a body-use activity.

4. Use Step 12 to visualize achieving your goal.

5. Consider trying to reduce rest times by cutting the length of the rest period by, say, a minute at a time, or exchange some of them for a relaxation session or exercises.

6. Make time for recording your progress and successes in your personal notebook.

7. Make time for family and friends—and, if possible, discuss your program with them to gain their understanding, support, and encouragement.

# UNIT 8

■

# Enjoying Yourself

## CONTENTS

# Enjoying Yourself

"Feel-good" endorphins are produced in our bodies when we are relaxed, focused, and happy. These endorphins are our bodies' own natural painkillers and so when we are engaged in enjoyable activities, we not only gain in pleasure but we also allow our natural healing processes to flow. Despite our physical difficulties, we can still enjoy pleasurable activities in our lives. In fact, the very reason we need to make sure we *do* find time to enjoy life is because we have pain.

When your body first started to hurt, you may have altered your lifestyle in order to cope with the discomfort, and, in your preoccupation with trying to cope with the pain, you may very well have forgotten to take time out for enjoyment. Enjoying yourself is not a luxury or self-indulgence. The personal self-expression and creativity we all gain from enjoying our pastimes is one of the most important aspects of our lives. Our interests and hobbies give us lasting satisfaction, making us more rounded, fully developed people; we think more positively and our stress levels become lowered. Best of all, enjoyable activities distract us from pain; we can, after all, only think about one thing at a time. Take some time, or make some time, to work through the steps in this unit and plan a campaign of action that will help you to add enjoyment to your life and move the focus of attention from pain to pleasure. By consistently changing this focus, you alter your whole perception of life, and of the pain, and become a happier person. Developing strong pleasure pathways in your brain goes a long way to overcoming the pain pathways.

# STEP 1: WHAT DO YOU ENJOY?

Find a time when you know you can be peaceful and undisturbed for about twenty minutes. If you find it difficult to set aside time just for yourself, explain to your family and friends that you need this quiet period to work on your campaign to care for and reduce your pain. Arrange to make this session really comfortable and full of pleasure. This time is for you, so spoil yourself. Indulge all your senses, the senses of smell, sight, sound, touch, and taste. To induce comfort, sensuality, and peace, try to include some of the elements below in the surroundings you choose.

A quiet and comfortable place to sit or lounge, outdoors or indoors
A sunny spot or a cool, shady area
Still or moving water
Trees and plants
Country views
The sound of birds
Fragrant flowers
Gentle music
Soft lights, candlelight
Air perfumed with essential oils

Arrange to have a few treats and your favorite drink on hand. Make this a special time in any way you can. It *is* special because it marks a new beginning for you.

We use a very simple method to find out what gives you enjoyment. This method enables you to contact your inner self, your inner wisdom, your intuition. We all have this inner sense of wisdom that knows instinctively what we need, what is good for us, and what is true for us. This intuitive sense is usually swamped by everyday busyness and so becomes neglected. By learning to listen quietly to the messages from our body and mind, we make contact with our real self. When we take time to make contact with it, this inner self is the source of great power and strength to us. With practice, you may find this method of connecting such a useful tool that you use it in many areas of your life, especially if you have a problem of any kind to solve.

You don't have to complete the whole exercise at one time; you can break off at the end of any one of the stages, if you prefer. You will need some sheets of plain paper and a pen or pencil. Unplug the telephone if there is no one else to answer it.

### Getting in Touch With Your Inner Self

*Before you pick up your writing materials, relax by allowing your breath to become slightly deeper and slower for a few moments. Then, as you breathe out, allow your face to relax, and smile gently. This will put you in a calmer, more reflective mood. . . . Then, quietly pick up your pen or pencil and, in the middle of your sheet of paper, draw a circle.*

*Inside the circle write:*

*And now, become very still. Let your mind relax and ask yourself the question in the circle, allowing your mind spontaneously to produce answers for you. Take note of the very first thought coming to your mind, as this is your true self speaking. Write the thought next to the circle, attached by a short line.*

*Now relax, then go back to the question and ask it again of yourself, once more writing down the first thought that comes. Keep asking yourself the question until no more answers surface. As you receive answers, jot them around the circle, in any order.*

You may collect yet more information by thinking back through your life, remembering everything you have ever enjoyed or found pleasurable. Note absolutely any experiences that have given you real happiness and made you feel good, whether or not they are part of your life now. They don't all have to be "doings"; make sure you list things appealing to your senses too—listening, watching, hearing, tasting, touching. Take as much time as you need for this.

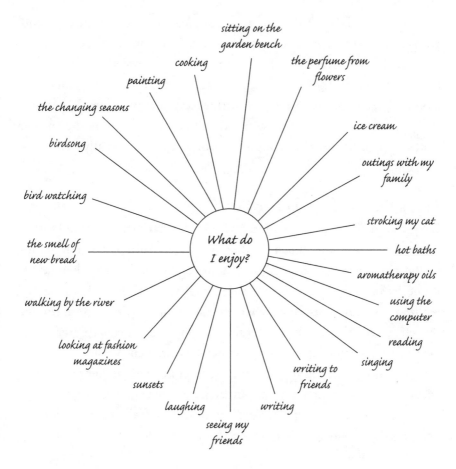

Your chart will look completely different from the example above, as it will reflect your pleasures.

## *Making Time for Enjoyment*

You will now have in front of you a page full of information about the ways you personally gain pleasure and enjoyment. This is the time to make a promise to yourself to take, or *make*, time each day to enjoy yourself, no matter how busy you are or how much pain you have. You aren't being idle, self-indulgent, lazy, or wasting time; making time for enjoyment is a vital part of learning to cope with and reduce your pain as well as enhancing your life. Your family and friends will also appreciate the new, more relaxed and happier you. So, ask yourself, early on in the day, *"What am I going to do to enjoy myself today?"* Choose an item from your list of activities and pleasures, set a time to spend with it, hold the activity in your mind until the time arrives, and then *enjoy* it. Do this every day. It doesn't have to be something major; we are talking more about simple pleasures. It is enough, sometimes, to stop and spend a few minutes savoring your surroundings, especially if you can involve nature in some way. Take time to enjoy the smells, tastes, sights, textures, and sounds around you, being really conscious of them.

### Lucy's Discoveries from Her Chart

Lucy found there were many activities on her chart she could enjoy immediately, without much further planning. Although her mobility in the garden is very limited, she decided she could grow her favorite herbs in pots indoors. Until she completed her chart, Lucy hadn't realized just how important it was to her to spend time just sitting in the garden soaking up the peaceful atmosphere. She plans to organize a new bed for perfumed flowers near her favorite bench. She loves writing and has determined to keep in closer contact with all her family and friends. As a reminder, Lucy has pinned a card on her fridge door headed *"Enjoyments—which ones today?"* with a list of all the activities she had jotted down around her circle.

### Your Turn Now

It is unlikely that many of the activities you have on your chart cost any money or require a lot of special planning. All it needs is for you to become aware of the benefits of setting aside some time every day, and then to make a pact with yourself to find space for one or more of your pleasurable activities. It doesn't matter whether it is for five minutes or fifty, as long as you keep to your promise. Be resolute in keeping this special time just for you to enjoy in whatever way gives you pleasure. Treat it as one of the most important things in your life. If it helps to remind you, make a list and pin it up where you will see it early in the day.

> *Every day . . .*
> - *First thing every morning ask yourself, "What can I do to enjoy myself today?"*

- *Read your list and add to it as more ideas surface.*
- *Do something from your list at least once a day.*
- *Congratulate yourself for bringing enjoyment into your life.*

## STEP 2: WHAT WOULD YOU *LIKE* TO DO?

Moving on from your current enjoyments, the next step is to discover a goal for an exciting new project to bring yet more pleasure into your life. This time you are going to find out which activities you would really like to do for your enjoyment if you ever had the time or opportunity. This could be something that is a lifetime ambition of yours, something you have always dreamed of doing one day.

Use the same method as in Step 1 to contact your inner self, that special true self that lives deep inside you. This part of you will always know what it is you truly need and desire. With the use of the circle to focus your attention, you can find out exactly what it is that would give you lasting satisfaction at a deep level. Again, you will need some sheets of plain paper and a pen or pencil.

*Before you begin, give yourself a few quiet moments and focus on your breath as it flows in and out of your body. Allow your breath to become slightly deeper and slower. As you breathe out, allow your face to relax, and smile gently. This will put you in a calmer, more reflective mood. . . . Then, quietly pick up your pen or pencil and, in the middle of your sheet of paper, draw a circle. Write in the middle of the circle:*

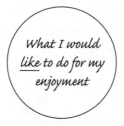

*Take the same approach as in Step 1. Relax, ask yourself the question, and let your intuition provide the answers. Make*

*a note of everything and anything you have always wanted to do, even if you think it may be rather difficult for you at the moment. This may give you ideas for another activity with which you could cope, or you may be able to come to the activity later on. Keep referring back to the question until you have exhausted all possible answers.*

Think of some of the things you always thought you would like to do if you ever had the time or space. You may remember some previous hobby or desire you had that you would like to try again; let your imagination run free. If you've always wanted to paint or sing, write it down. If writing or craftwork appeals to you, write it down. You want to find out what you *really* would like to do; you want to find out your dreams. It's for your eyes only, so open up and admit your long-held desires, no matter whether they are "ordinary" or more ambitious activities; all that matters is that they're special to *you*. You don't have to write anything to impress anyone else or to please anyone else; this is just for you. Your chart will look completely different from Lucy's chart, shown below, because it will reflect your interests and ambitions.

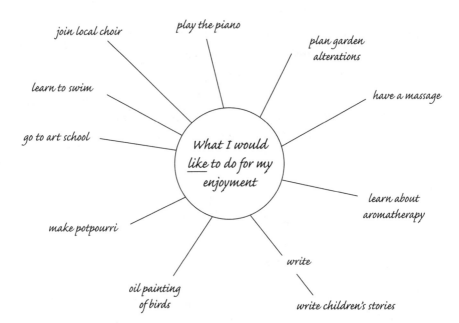

## STEP 3: GOAL SELECTING

You now have a page full of notes of pleasure-giving situations and another of activities you would like to do for your enjoyment. This information is your database for choosing an activity as your new goal. It may be something that had been just a dream but which you might now be able to realize, or an activity you may have neglected and could pick up again. The lists may very well lead you on to something new you had never even thought of before.

> *Take a really careful look at your notes and then ask a few questions to learn more about your real likes, pleasures, and ambitions. Ask questions like these (there are no right or wrong answers):*
>
>> *Do the situations that give you pleasure all fall into the same basic categories? For example, are they mainly:*
>>
>> *Social, involved with other people?*
>> *Practical, using materials or objects of some kind?*
>> *Reading or dealing with information in some way?*
>>
>> *If they are all similar, is there anything else you would like to do for a change or for balance in your life?*

Now, from your list, select just one activity to develop. In choosing, bear in mind your current situation and try to find something you could reasonably attain in small steps. You will be sure to find that your list has produced something within your scope.

## STEP 4: ACHIEVING YOUR GOAL

> *Having selected your goal, write it in the center of another circle on a big sheet of plain paper. It is important to make the goal a clear, precise statement of what you want to achieve, such as "I want to paint with watercolors" or "I want to go to the club every week."*
>
> *Next, jot around the circle everything that comes to mind*

*that you need to do to achieve your goal. This way you will know exactly what is going to be involved. By breaking the goal into separate steps, you will be able successfully to accomplish your aim. Each step is an achievement for you, and so remember to congratulate yourself as you progress.*

*You may need to break each step into more stages of its own; connect them with lines as in the example on page 151. Make separate lists for some of the steps if the page begins to fill up. Ask yourself what you will need to achieve each step. Ask "When?" "Where?" "How?" types of questions at each step. For example:*

> *If you need to get books for reference, how will you get them?*
>
> *Where will you get them from?*
> *When will you be able to do this?*
>
> *Is there anything within this activity too painful for you to do now?*
>
> *What is your current pain tolerance for this activity?*
> *Can you improve this in any way?*
>
> *When you have found your starting point, when can you start?*

Lucy examined her notes very carefully and concluded that she wanted to concentrate on writing stories for children. She would need to ask some friends to help her obtain books, and the typing would have to be done in short bursts, as she was unable to sit for very long. Lucy thought she could use her resting times to make notes and then type them up later. She was keen to start and planned to begin straight away by making a few notes for her first story.

Look at the chart on the facing page to see how Lucy worked out her writing activities. This is an example only; what you want to do will probably be completely different. Your charts and ambitions will be yours alone, reflecting your own special interests.

You may find that it takes you a long time to go through all the stages toward achieving your goal, but never give up. Remember Hare and Tortoise in their race? "Slow and steady" won the race. Don't lose sight of your aim and make sure every step is well within your capabilities; *enjoy* each step for itself. If you find you have taken too much on board, drop back to a more reasonable level and then build up again more carefully.

When this first goal is completed, or well under way, you may want to embark upon another. By using the circle method to contact your inner wisdom, you now know how to ensure success.

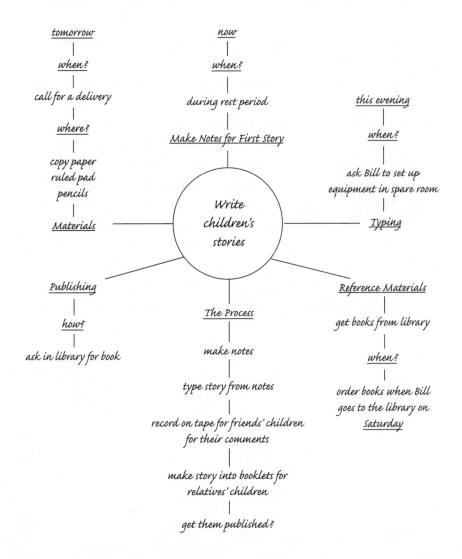

## ACTION GUIDELINES

1. The most important aspect of this unit is learning to focus on having enjoyment in your life in order to strengthen the pleasure pathways in your mind. Never let go of your goal, no matter how long it may take to achieve it.

2. Find the starting point for your new goal and begin immediately by setting aside a short time each day for your activity. The time allocation will reflect whatever is reasonable for your physical ability and your pain level. If it is only a few minutes, that's fine; if it's an hour, that's also fine. Make it a priority to do something toward your goal every day without fail.

3. In addition, choose something from your "enjoyment activities" lists at least once a day.

4. *First thing every morning ask yourself "What can I do to* ENJOY *myself today?" Do this* EVERY DAY.

5. Develop your relationship with your inner self. This wise part of you is always available to you to consult in moments of need. You can ask questions of your inner wisdom, such as, "What do I need in this situation?" "What am I feeling about this situation?" "What do I want?" "How can I help my body to recover?" or any other question that is relevant to you at any time. You may not always receive an answer instantly, but the answer will surely come, perhaps during the day or even some days later. You will know when you have an answer because you will have a feeling of, "Of course! I understand," as though a light has been switched on inside you.

# UNIT 9

■

# Flare-Ups

## CONTENTS

# Flare-Ups

S etbacks or flare-ups of symptoms do occur from time to time, your body telling you in no uncertain terms that it needs even more care and attention than usual. Flare-up time is when you need especially to have an attitude of loving-kindness and compassion toward yourself, plus well-planned strategies for coping with the situation. If you have a flare-up at the moment, even if you haven't yet read and used the techniques in the rest of the book, you will find ideas here to help you to cope with your situation now and a structure for dealing with possible flare-ups in the future. Flare-ups are over faster and are more easily dealt with if you know what to do beforehand to steer into calmer waters once again.

## THE FLARE-UP ACTION PLAN

A setback or flare-up can occur very quickly, perhaps as the result of overdoing things, an accident, or an illness; or it can arise gradually and you may notice only that you're having difficulty coping with your activities after a period of time. As soon as you do become aware that you are in a flare-up situation, you need to begin a Flare-Up Action Plan to sustain and nurture yourself and to ensure that you come out stronger and more resilient at the end. There are many wonderful techniques available to you for easing your discomfort and keeping your spirits high and positive during a flare-up. This is the time to use all those skills you may already have acquired and, later on in the flare-up when you are feeling a little more comfortable, to investigate some new techniques.

A flare-up is not something you now face alone. Use this book as a friend and guide to uplift and sustain you on your way, and know that my thoughts are with you wherever you are.

## STEP 1: STOP

*Face it—immediately* STOP *what you are doing and thinking, take control, and decide to* CHANGE *to your Flare-Up Action Plan.*

As soon as you become aware that your body is not happy and it is telling you so in very strong terms, you reach a choice point. You can choose to continue as you are or you can STOP and CHANGE direction and begin to put your Flare-Up Action Plan into effect. Therefore, as soon as you realize that you're in a flare-up situation, the first, and most important, thing for you to do is to *face the flare-up* and decide to *take charge* of the situation. It is as though the path you are on has reached a fork, signposted one way CONTINUE AS YOU ARE and the other way FLARE-UP ACTION PLAN. When you make the decision to turn on to the Flare-Up Action Plan path, it acts like a switch inside you; you immediately switch off any sense of helplessness and switch on positive feelings of being in charge and in control. Your feelings are suddenly transformed; you feel different about the situation. The improvement comes because you have faced the situation and brought in a constructive attitude—*you* are in charge again and you are willing to find ways to help yourself.

So, when your thoughts are tumbling about and you are feeling the force of the flare-up symptoms, the very first action for you to take is to say

"STOP"

to yourself; see it as though it was a Stop sign at the fork in the road we talked about earlier. You can say "STOP" either out loud or inside your head, but you need to say it very firmly and convincingly in order to impress the message upon your subconscious mind (more about your subconscious mind and positive inner talk later). "STOP" means stopping everything—what you are thinking, what you are doing. Just saying a firm "STOP" will shock your mind into a few moments of blessed silence. The space you have created in your mind only lasts for a split second. Capitalize upon this moment's grace; it enables you to CHANGE direction from the road you have been traveling on. To travel on the new road, you need quickly to fill the space created in your mind with new, constructive thoughts to ensure that there is no room for any negative self-talk to flood in again.

*Use the positive thoughts from the list of affirmations below to ease this first step of the Flare-Up Action Plan. Repeat the sentences over and over to yourself wholeheartedly and with real conviction, affirming that you are in charge of the situation:*

> *First . . .*      STOP
> *Then affirm . . .* "*I know what to do.*"
> "*I am in charge here.*"
> "*I can cope with this if I use the strategies in the Flare-Up Action Plan.*"

## STEP 2: DIAPHRAGMATIC BREATHING AND AFFIRMATIONS

*Use deep diaphragmatic breathing combined with affirmations for natural pain relief and a calm and positive mind.*

Having gained initial control of the situation and of those negative thoughts, it is essential that you remain in control. Now is the time to concentrate upon directing your next action. You are now going to focus on deep, diaphragmatic breathing, as this is the key to all natural pain relief and, later on, the basis of relaxation and meditation practices.

Diaphragmatic breathing will help to relieve tension in your muscles; it will relax your mind and allow your body's own painkillers, endorphins, to flow. This is how to focus on diaphragmatic breathing:

*Make yourself as comfortable as you can, wherever you are, standing, sitting, or lying down. Make sure your clothing is loose around your middle. Breathing through your nose, take your attention to your abdomen and just observe it for a moment or two as it rises and falls with the inflow and outflow of your breath. Allow your shoulders to drop. On your next out breath, open your mouth, then let the breath out with a sigh, out loud. Let the breath out right down to your abdomen like this . . . "Aaaaaaaahhhhhhhhhhhh." . . . Just let everything go. . . . Try a slight smile at the same time; this will relax all the muscles of your face and send positive messages to your subconscious mind. Don't force anything, be gentle.*

*On your next out breath, sigh again, this time letting the sigh go from the top of your head right down through your body and out through the bottom of your feet. There's no need to push or strain. The out breath can be longer than the in breath. Taking the in breath need not concern you; it will take care of itself.*

*After these two lovely releasing breaths, you can now just allow your breath to come quietly and easily. Notice how your breathing has become slower and deeper. Notice your lower ribs expand and contract at the front, back, and sides. Check to see if your shoulders are still dropped and relaxed. Continue by paying attention to five or six of these natural, peaceful breaths. This is diaphragmatic, or abdominal, breathing. (See Unit 1 for further information.)*

Guide and support yourself over the intense stage of the flare-up by repeating some affirmations over and over to yourself, out loud if you like, to reinforce their positive impact.

*Choose from this selection of reassuring and instructive affirmations, or make up similar ones of your own. Repeat them quietly and calmly to yourself, either inside your head or aloud.*

*"I concentrate on my breathing."*
*"Be peaceful . . . be still."*
*"Relax . . . this will pass."*
*"Breathe out . . . and let go. . . . "*
*"My breathing is slow and steady."*
*"I let go, I float and flow with it."*

*"I take one moment at a time and concentrate on what I am doing now."*

*"I let go thoughts of the past and the future."*

*"I breathe in relaxation and healing energy."*

*[On in breath] "I breathe in and relax. . . . [On out breath] I breathe out and let go. . . ."*

*"I breathe into the sensations and I soften my body."*

*"I allow the sensations to float around me."*

*"With encouraging and positive thoughts, I can achieve wonders."*

*or simply,*

*"Peace," "Relax," or any other comforting word.*

*If the sensations from your body are very intense, you may find it preferable to choose just one affirmation that particularly resonates with you. Keep repeating it again and again until the sensations alter or subside. At the height of the flare-up, you may, alternatively, want to concentrate on the rhythm of your breathing alone.*

Check your breathing throughout the day to ensure that you're breathing in this deep and natural way.

Continue to use encouraging, supporting affirmations throughout the flare-up. The way you view the flare-up and what you tell yourself make all the difference to your progress. It is natural and understandable that negative thoughts enter your mind at this time, but it is not helpful for you to dwell upon them. Throughout this book there are dynamic and mood-raising affirmations from which you can select a short list or use as ideas for making up your own. It is helpful to write them on small reminder cards to keep near you. Repeat the words over and over many times during the day, either out loud or inside your head. Say them in a wholehearted manner with real meaning to the words, even if you don't think or feel that way at the moment. You are not deceiving yourself; you are directing yourself. The affirmations point the way for you to move, rather like instructions. (More about affirmations in Unit 2.)

*If negative thoughts reappear at any time during the flare-up, stop*
*them in their tracks by immediately returning to Steps 1 and 2 of*
*the Flare-Up Action Plan.*

### SUMMARY OF STEPS 1 AND 2

**Step 1**

- Face it—immediately say "STOP" to what you're doing and thinking.
- Take control and decide to CHANGE to your Flare-Up Action Plan.

*"I know what to do."*

**Step 2**

- Use deep diaphragmatic breathing combined with affirmations for natural pain relief and a calm and positive mind.

*"I concentrate on my breathing."*

# STEP 3: SELECT YOUR NEXT STRATEGY

*Once you are back in control of the situation with steady,*
*calming breathing and some reassuring affirmations, you leave*
*yourself free to concentrate upon your other supporting*
*and nourishing strategies.*

The ideas in Step 3 are not in any particular order, although relaxation makes an excellent beginning to your Flare-Up Action Plan, and Pacing Yourself, which comes later in this unit, is best taken on board early on in the flare-up. Look through the ideas in Step 3 and select the techniques that particularly appeal to you. You may find that some techniques are more effective for you than others at different stages of the flare-up. There is no *right* way to comfort and support yourself during a flare-up, so use whatever helps *you*.

## Relaxation
(See Unit 1 for further ideas.)
The diaphragmatic breathing method in Step 2 leads quite naturally to the relaxation process itself. For the session, sit or lie down and relax

completely for fifteen to twenty minutes, entering a deeply peaceful and relaxed state of body and mind. During flare-up time, when your body is in greater need than usual, treat yourself to as many relaxation sessions as you can during the day; deep breathing and relaxation are the keys to effective natural pain control.

Relaxation will calm you and, as you let go of any tension, give you some relief from the painful sensations. When you relax deeply, you not only release tight muscles, but you also sometimes release emotions and thoughts you have been holding on to, perhaps feelings of sadness about the flare-up. If this happens, allow these thoughts and feelings to come to the surface and let them go. Once they arise and are experienced, they are released and finished with. Be grateful for this opportunity of releasing inner tension. Continue with your relaxation practice, as ultimately it is one of the most vital factors in reducing and coping with pain. Add some affirmations for a reassuring input of positive thoughts.

## Golden Light Relaxation

Try this lovely Golden Light Relaxation as your next strategy in the Flare-Up Action Plan. It will give your body and mind peace and comfort and allow your natural healing energy to flow. Take your time and, where there are dots, leave pauses to enjoy the relaxation. You could, of course, make a recording of the script yourself or ask someone to read it for you, but for maximum benefit, listen to the lovely version of this relaxation on the accompanying CD. If you choose to just listen to the CD, it will still be helpful to read through the following script.

> *Find a quiet place and take off your shoes and loosen any tight clothing. Lie down where you can be comfortable and warm. Make sure you won't be disturbed for about twenty minutes. Take a few moments to allow your body to soften and relax down into the surface beneath you. . . .*
>
> *Take your attention to your breath and, breathing through your nose, just observe it for a moment or so as it flows in and out. There's no need to strain; natural deep breathing takes place quietly and effortlessly. There's no need to do anything except to notice how your breathing is becoming slower and deeper.*

*Notice how still you are becoming and how quiet your body is
apart from the gentle rise and fall of your abdomen. . . .*

*With each breath, you spread warmth and soothing relaxation
all around your body. . . . And so travel in your mind around your
body, becoming aware of each part in turn . . . and as you do so,
allow it to soften and release even more. . . . Feel each part become
yet more comfortable and warm . . . relaxing your neck . . . your
head . . . your face, which is cool and calm . . . your shoulders,
which relax and sink down into the surface beneath them . . . your
arms . . . your hands . . . your back . . . your abdomen . . . your
legs. Feel how heavy your legs are . . . and your feet.*

*And now, as you breathe in, imagine that you also breathe
in a beautiful soft golden light. . . . Your breath takes the light
right around your body . . . and your whole body becomes filled
with this golden healing light. . . . Take your mind to any area
that needs special attention and see the light flowing to the
area, bathing it with gentle, soothing relaxation and more
peaceful comfort. . . . Your body's own natural healing power is
energized by the relaxation. . . .*

*Imagine there is so much golden healing light in your body
that it overflows and you are also surrounded with this beautiful
light, like a golden glowing aura all the way around your body.
. . . And now your whole body is being soothed and nourished,
on both the inside and the outside. . . . You breathe in golden
healing light . . . and breathe out golden healing light. . . . Take
a few more moments to enjoy the comfort and peace you have
created . . . and then take these feelings back with you as you
slowly and gradually become aware of the surface beneath you,
and, when you are ready, come back to the room. . . . Lie quietly
for a few moments and enjoy the peace that is always within you
. . . and remember, you can regain this feeling at any time you
want; it is always there for you. . . . [long pause] . . .*

*Your own healing powers are now at work and all is well.*

*Know that every time you relax in this deep way you are
maximizing your natural healing powers.*

*When you are ready, stretch your fingers and toes . . . feel peaceful and calm, yet alert and ready to go about your day, taking these relaxed feelings with you.*

Use this relaxation method at least once every day, more often if you can when your body needs extra care and loving attention.

## Relaxation and Affirmations

One of my favorite ways to relax is to use a method that happily combines affirmation techniques with relaxation. This next technique makes for a lovely relaxation because it is simple and totally adaptable. The rhythm and pattern of the words are very repetitive and comforting and are ideally soporific when used last thing at night for slipping into a peaceful sleep.

*Talk, in your mind, to different parts of your body, allowing them to relax and let go in turn. The following list is an example of the words you could use, but you should choose words that resonate with you. For example, instead of "peaceful and calm" you could use "heavy and warm" or "soft and loose."*

> *My left toes are peaceful,*
> *My left toes are peaceful and calm,*
> *My left toes are letting go.*
>
> *My right toes are peaceful,*
> *My right toes are peaceful and calm,*
> *My right toes are letting go.*
>
> *My left foot is peaceful,*
> *My left foot is peaceful and calm,*
> *My left foot is letting go.*
>
> *My right foot . . . [etc.]*

*Using the same format, travel in your mind, talking about your ankles, calves, knees, thighs, pelvis, all around your abdomen, up your back, to your shoulders, down your arms and hands, then your neck and head. Include any parts of your body needing special attention and spend some extra time in those areas. You*

*can also include your "insides" too, if you like: your heart, stom-*
*ach, for example. I like to finish with:*

> *"My mind is peaceful,*
> *My mind is peaceful and calm,*
> *My mind is letting go.*

> *"My feelings are peaceful,*
> *My feelings are peaceful and calm,*
> *My feelings are letting go.*

> *"All within me is peaceful and calm,*
> *The air around me is peaceful and calm,*
> *I am at one with all and everything."*

As mentioned previously, this relaxation is wonderfully helpful if it is used to calm and relax you at bedtime. However, if you wake in the night or still find difficulty with sleeping, do get up after twenty minutes or so to break the pattern of not sleeping. Don't try to analyze the situation; accept it as it is. Say "STOP" to negative thoughts and repeat to yourself, *"Tomorrow* is for thinking. I put away my worries and concerns till then. Now is for *feeling."* Walk about, stretch, or do something peacefully for a short while and then return to bed and *feel* your way through the relaxation again, not thinking but instead concentrating your attention on feeling the different parts of your body.

Here are some suggestions for affirmations to use throughout the day or at the relaxation time.

> *"I set aside time each day for relaxation."*
> *"I am peaceful and calm."*
> *"It is easy for me to relax."*
> *"When I relax, I let go of all my cares."*
> *"I relax and let go . . . it's a wonderful feeling."*
> *"When I relax, I allow my healing processes to flow."*
> *"I am taking care of myself in a deep and nourishing way."*
> *"I sleep peacefully right through the night."*

## Meditation

(See Unit 6 for further details.)

Although meditation and relaxation have some similarities, in that we usually sit or lie down for a period of time and enter a different state of mind, they have very different aims. We can perhaps regard relaxation as going away on holiday and meditation more as a coming home. During relaxation, we usually escape from whatever we are doing and thinking throughout the day. When we are meditating, we deliberately stay very aware of what is going on around us, as well as coming home to our true inner self, where we find a timeless space. We can use both relaxation and meditation methods on different occasions during the day or we may choose to use one of these skills only.

Meditation is best carried out in an upright sitting position but can be done in any position you find comfortable—but not so comfortable that you fall asleep. The aim of meditation is to stay awake and aware, yet maintain a relaxed poise while you become as one again with your true inner self. The simplest way to meditate is to place your attention on your breath and "watch" it as it goes in and out of your body. When your mind wanders, as it will, gently bring it back to observing your breath again.

When you practice meditation, you will have the means to help you to get through trying occasions when you may be wondering, "What will happen?" "How will I cope?" "When will it end?" By training yourself to be totally present *now*, all you have to deal with is *now*, and that much is bearable. It will help you to cope with *this* moment—which you can—and *this* moment . . . and *this* moment . . . and not to concern yourself with thoughts of the future of the pain or of how you were in the past before the pain.

When we meditate with the pain, we can breathe into the sensation itself and watch the pain as it changes, being sometimes here, sometimes gone. The pain floats around us as we go deeper into meditation, and somehow it is no longer "us" or a pain, but just a sensation "out there" somewhere. This, for me, is the most effective way to cope with the pain.

This kind of approach is what we mean by being patient. Patience means living in the here and now, not with half of ourselves stretched toward tomorrow and the other half lingering in the past. When we live our lives in the present, we give ourselves the time to enjoy and appreciate many things around us in our world. When we do this, we may well find that the pain retreats or even disappears. We need to be kind to ourselves, to slow down, to let time flow by us and not fret about things we feel committed to do. We need a holiday from pressure and to let things go for a while until we have our energy back. Our focus needs to be on ways in which to help ourselves and on what we *can* do at this moment. The practice of meditation can achieve all of this for us. It is a way of being in touch with ourselves in a deep and loving way.

Add some of these affirmations to your list. Repeat them often during the day or even during the meditation.

> *"Peace, be still."*
> *"I can go to this inner center of peace and calm at any time. It is always there for me."*
> *"My center is still and peaceful."*
> *"I live my life moment by moment."*
> *"I can accept and bear this moment . . . and this . . . and this . . . and this is all that matters."*
> *"When the sensations are at their most intense, I talk myself through, concentrating carefully on one thing at a time."* (For example, *"First I pick up my cup, I look at the pattern on the cup, I bring the cup to my lips. . . ."*)
> *"I breathe into the sensation."*

### Visualization

(See Unit 4 for further ideas.)

Visualization is a powerful tool because it can effect changes in your body and so is a therapy in itself. Through using visualization in a positive way, you can activate your healing systems and make real changes in your body.

The creative side of your mind needs to be allowed to come alive before starting a visualization, so always spend some time relaxing first, as this allows your imaginative mind to open. You can use visualization skills in many ways to help your body. You can ease the pain by imagining you are standing in a cool waterfall or lying on a delightful bed of soft, fluffy clouds. Or, in your imagination you can change the pain to a form more acceptable to you—for example, turning a large hot red ball of sensation into a tiny cool blue ball. With practice, the sensation may even disappear altogether.

In your imagination, try transferring the pain into the shape of a ball just outside your body. Use your mind to reduce the size of the ball just slightly, perhaps from a tennis-ball size to a golf-ball size, then reduce it again if you can. Once you have reduced the pain as much as you are able to at this time, return the new size to your body. Again, you may be able to reduce the pain until it is gone. This exercise will build your confidence in controlling the pain.

Another way to use visualization is to take yourself off on an imaginary adventure: to woody glades, beautiful gardens, tropical sands, or floating away in a balloon basket. This type of visualization relaxes and refreshes you. Always, at the end of the session, see yourself smiling and being full of health and vigor. This will send positive messages to your body and mind.

Try this visualization to mend a part of your body. With relaxed concentration, you can influence and allow your body to make subtle shifts toward healing. You can read through the visualization and then practice it while you are relaxing, record the visualization yourself, or ask someone to read it to you. Where you see dots, leave plenty of time to allow your imagination to range free.

*Find a comfortable, quiet place where you can relax and be peaceful. . . . Place your attention on the inflow and outflow of your breath. . . . Begin to feel peaceful and calm. . . . On your next out breath, let all the breath out with a slight sigh . . . aaahhhh. . . . Let your face relax . . . and allow yourself a half smile. . . . On the next out breath, let the sigh go all the way from the top of your head to the soles of your feet. . . . Your body is soft . . . your mind is peaceful . . . you feel totally relaxed. . . . And now, imagine that you become very, very tiny . . . as light as thistledown . . . and float down inside yourself*

*until you are near the place in your body needing special atten-*
*tion. . . . See the area as you imagine it to be at the moment. . . .*
*It doesn't matter if you don't know all the medical details; your*
*own ideas are far more important on this occasion. . . . Just*
*sense how it appears to you. . . . Get a really clear picture of*
*how it seems . . . the structures, the shapes, colors, textures,*
*and even the sounds involved. . . . [longer pause] . . . Now set*
*about repairing and mending the part. . . . Do whatever needs*
*to be done to make it as good as new. . . . You may want to*
*cleanse the area using a foam spray or springwater . . . or you*
*may want to accept assistance from others, perhaps little drag-*
*ons breathing fire to cleanse the area . . . or perhaps use an iron*
*to smooth out creases and bumps. . . . You could protect and*
*support an area with tiny downy pillows . . . then soothe the*
*area with wonderful healing gels and lotions. . . . Create in your*
*imagination whatever you feel you need for the task. . . . See*
*your tiny self being very busy, very strong, yet gentle and able*
*to achieve wonders. . . . Be really creative and inventive, use*
*pictures and images that appeal to you. . . . [longer pause] . . .*

*You may ask yourself, "What does my body need?" . . . and*
*wait for ideas to spring into your mind. . . . Keep going; spend*
*as long as you need here inside yourself to make the area whole*
*and perfect.*

*When the area has been cleansed and repaired and is work-*
*ing efficiently and healthily, look around and feel proud of the*
*work you have done. . . . Take plenty of time with this stage:*
*see the area shining and gleaming with good health. . . . Then*
*slowly and gently return to your normal size. . . . And then,*
*when you are ready, come back to the room. . . . Carry on with*
*your day, knowing that you have made a difference as to how*
*your body is working and that you have given freedom to your*
*healing process.*

Here are some affirmations you may want to repeat during the day to
encourage the imaginative side of your mind to flourish:

*"When I relax, I free my imagination."*

*"My creative mind works wonders for me."*

*"I make use of my inner strengths and imaginative powers."*

*"I already have within me all I need to release pain and allow my healing processes to flow."*

### Releasing Your Feelings

(See Unit 5 for further ideas.)

When we have a flare-up, it is quite likely and understandable that we feel emotionally upset. These negative feelings are perfectly okay provided we don't bottle them up. Feelings are for *feeling* and need to be expressed and let go. We need to take time to deal with any feelings we may be suppressing, or those we may be expressing inappropriately, such as being irritable with others, when in truth we are angry about the pain. When we release our emotions in an appropriate way, we enable our healing process to continue smoothly. If this is your need, try the following technique to clear emotional blockages. When you are quiet and receptive, you become open to your intuitive, wise self.

*Spend a few moments allowing your breath to become calm and deep and then ask,*

"What am I feeling about this pain?"

*Answers will be in the form of the very first thoughts coming into your consciousness, a picture or a sensation in your body, or just a feeling of some kind, a knowing. If you receive an answer along the lines of "sad" or "angry" or some other negative emotion, you can then ask yourself,*

"What can I learn from this that will release me from this emotion?"

*Keep asking this question until you have a feeling of "that's it," or "I understand." You can then ask yourself,*

"Is there any action I could take?"

*This process will help to clear any emotional blockages and give*
*you a lead for action you could take.*

You can also physically release emotion with, say, crying if you are sad or thumping a pillow to release angry feelings. Sharing emotions, telling others how you feel, can also help you to understand and release them. If this is not convenient, you can write them down, expressing just how you feel on to the paper. At the completion, when the emotion has gone, destroy the paper without reading what is written. Move on as quickly as you can to take some action that will encourage more positive feelings.

### *Encouraging Positive Emotions*
(See Unit 3 for further ideas.)

It is essential for our progress that we do all we can to improve the way we feel and give ourselves much needed support, by deliberately fostering a positive attitude. We can do this by focusing on what we *can* do and what we do have. When we recognize these positive aspects of our lives, we feel more secure and in balance. Release all thoughts or regrets about what you cannot do for the moment. Whatever your situation, there is still plenty you can appreciate and for which you can be thankful.

Physically changing our expression will also help to pull us away from negativity. When we smile, we communicate a strong message to our subconscious mind that says, "All is well; relax and be content." We don't even have to feel like smiling for this to happen. If we relax our facial muscles deliberately and allow our lips to be upturned into a gentle half smile, that same message will be sent regardless of our current feelings. Amazingly, we very soon become more relaxed and serene as the message is received by our mind and body. A good way to try the smile therapy is to place your attention on your breath as you inhale and exhale, allowing your face to relax and half smile. Practice while you are listening to the radio, to music, looking out of the window, or, indeed, during any other activity.

Take every opportunity to watch and listen to laughter-making films, radio programs, or tapes and CDs or to rerun in your mind amusing events from your life. Read humorous books, cartoons, or comics: they will all trigger the same response from your feel-good endorphins, which will improve your mood and reduce the pain.

Other blues-beaters are getting out for some physical activity if you can, chatting with friends, stroking an animal, treating yourself to a favorite meal or snack, getting close to nature, sitting in the sun for a short while, curling up with a special chocolate treat, planning an activity for when you are feeling better, listening to some favorite music, particularly if you can sing along with it. My favorite way to spoil myself is to have a hot relaxing bath in which I drop some special essential oils. I listen to some rhythm-and-blues music, which I accompany by what I call "body music"—I clap the rhythms of the songs all over my arms and legs, I play the rhythms in the water, in the air, on the side of the bath, finding different sounds from all the various surfaces; it's great fun and a guaranteed pick-me-up.

Here are a few affirmations for your emotional well-being—repeat them over and over until they feel true for you:

*"I am safe and secure and all is well."*
*"I have the power and authority in my life to release the past and accept my good now."*
*"I have so many blessings in my life."*
*"I love and approve of myself."*
*"I am happy to be me."*
*"I smile gently and feel serene."*
*"All is well in my world."*

### Accepting the Situation

Our attitude toward the flare-up can make a critical difference as to how well we cope with it and how smoothly we come through it. Just as one accepts the fall of the dice in a game, complete and utter acceptance of the situation is the way. We need to move on from the past and come into the present, saving our emotional and mental energies for dealing with the flare-up. We do this by accepting that the flare-up has happened and nothing can be gained by blaming anyone or anything, especially ourselves. The physical sensations *will* settle in their own time and we can help our body to quiet by having as peaceful and constructive an attitude as possible so that our natural healing process can take place efficiently and effectively. When we accept the situation, we are freeing ourselves from discouraging thoughts, all "If only . . ." type of thoughts, all thoughts of fighting the situation. It is as it is; it has happened, therefore no blaming, no regrets. Go with it, flow with it, don't fight it, allow it to take its course. Let it be. Acceptance means neither that we *like* the situation nor that we are giving in to it or are resigned to it: it merely acknowledges reality—what *is*. We are saying we can accept that the flare-up is here and that we are free now to continue with thinking about what needs to be done.

If you find unhelpful thoughts and feelings returning, repeat the STOP procedure in Step 1 and reinforce an attitude of acceptance with some positive inner talk, which will enable you to move on to one of your coping strategies again. Here are some ideas for affirmations to encourage an attitude of acceptance. Repeat them often during the day with an inner voice of quiet, calm conviction:

> *"Okay, it's happened: now I concentrate on what I do about it."*
> *"I accept the situation . . . I go with it. . . ."*
> *"I release thoughts of the past, which has gone, and the future, which is yet to come."*
> *"I will take one day at a time and concentrate on what I am doing now."*
> *"I accept the negative feelings and thoughts and let them pass through my mind without spending time on them. I let them go."*
> *"I am patient and I let time pass."*
> *"I let things take their course."*
> *"I allow whatever is happening to happen."*
> *"I let go, float and flow with it."*
> *"When I accept the situation, I free my energy to attend to what needs to be done."*

### Forgiveness

Our emotions are often heightened when we have a flare-up of pain and we may find that, in order to have a sense of feeling whole and to be able to move on, we need to have an attitude of forgiveness toward someone or something in our life. This can be a challenging thought and so we have to approach and support ourselves with understanding and compassion. We are the primary beneficiaries when we forgive either ourselves or someone else, because the act of forgiveness sets us free. Forgiveness does not imply a liking or condoning of the person or act involved: it is a process of letting go, allowing the past to stay where it belongs. The act of forgiveness leaves us free to live our life in the present and able to make progress. When we want to forgive, all we have to do is have the *desire* to forgive; it is as straightforward as that. Try the following visualization after a relaxation session when you are feeling peaceful and calm:

> *Relax and be still. . . . Have love within your heart. . . . When you are ready, ask yourself,* "Who or what is it I need to forgive?" *. . . The answer may come as a thought, a word, a picture, or a sensation of some sort. Go gently and take your time. . . . When you have the answer, imagine a distant hill, far away. . . . On the hill is a beautifully colored balloon with a wicker basket underneath. . . . On the balloon there is* FORGIVE *written in large gold letters. . . . See the person or people involved as being small enough to put in the basket. . . . With understanding, compassion, and a desire to forgive within you, say to them,* "I am willing to forgive you, I let you go." *. . . As you say this, imagine the balloon basket and the word* FORGIVE *floating gently away in the sky . . . gradually getting smaller and smaller and slowly disappearing out of sight.*
>
> *You may find that it is yourself you need to forgive; perhaps you have been blaming yourself or having other negative feelings about your situation. If this is so, place the whole emotion in the basket of the balloon . . . and this time say,* "I am willing to forgive myself, I let it go," *. . . and watch the balloon and the basket slowly, slowly float far, far away until they become a tiny speck . . . and then are gone. . . . As the balloon floats away, feel the negative emotions diminish and then disappear.*
>
> *Very, very slowly and gently bring yourself back to your room, feeling the peace and freedom within you.*

This is a beautiful exercise to repeat over and over. It will always feel releasing and give a sense of freedom because forgiving is an act of love that allows your heart to open as the hurts from the past disappear.

These are some affirmations to enhance the act of forgiveness. Use them often during the day or during the visualization.

> *"I forgive and let go."*
> *"I release anything that is not love from my life."*
> *"Harmony and peace fill my life."*
> *"I am filled with joy."*
> *"I am free of the past."*
> *"All is well in my world."*

### Pacing Yourself

(See Unit 7 for further details.)

When you have a setback or a flare-up of pain, your body is telling you it needs your attention and that it is finding it too difficult to carry on doing all the things you are asking it to do. When you pay attention to those messages from your body, you can allow it the respite it needs. Instead of expending energy on rushing around, your body can slow down and concentrate its energies on the healing process. No matter how many people you think are relying on you, or how many things you think you need to do, at this time it is essential that you put your body first in order to be able to allow it to regain health and strength. It's time to say "No, I'm sorry I can't do that today" if you are asked to do something you really aren't up to. You can also say the same thing to *yourself* when you think you have to do something, or want to do something that it would be sensible not to do just at the moment. When I find myself drawn toward doing something extra, I sometimes ask myself, "Will this be helping my back?" The answer is rarely yes!

I know how difficult it can be to let go and leave jobs and activities undone, but at flare-up times you need to treat yourself as you would treat a small child who needs care and support. You need to respect and nurture yourself and allow plenty of time to recover fully again. This may involve having to ask for extra help from family and friends where you can. Sometimes you may need to consider getting extra help from professional sources or from private care support systems. If so, let go of preconceived ideas and pride, and accept the support you need in order to become well again.

## Pacing at the Onset of a Flare-Up

In the first stage of a flare-up, *slow down,* and plan your day so you have many breaks from activity. Remember, your primary concern is your body's needs, and so it is essential to cut your sitting, standing, walking, and other activities to a level with which you can cope. This may mean reducing activities to about a half or a third of what you were doing before. Sometimes you may even decide that you need to rest completely for a day or so—use your own judgment here. However, it is still important to continue to move as much as possible, because unused muscles soon become stiff and sore. Do what you can, even if it's only half a minute at a time for the moment.

## Pacing at the End of a Flare-Up

It is relatively easy to take care of yourself when flare-up sensations are at their height, there often being little choice in the matter if your body demands complete rest. As you begin to recover and things start to become a little easier to handle as the flare-up subsides, the natural tendency is to be so thankful that you ease up on your vigilance and do much more, trying to catch up to make good the lost time. Instead of diving into those jobs that seem to be saying to you "I've *got* to be done now," be glad you're not in such pain and *enjoy* the extra resting time you have and the freedom from pressure. Don't rush back to work or start doing household jobs just yet. Give yourself as much time as you possibly can so the maximum amount of energy can go into healing your body.

Use the time for pleasurable activities to distract you from the remaining symptoms. It is also good to use this time as a revision and learning period; perhaps you could work through some of the units in this book, making a list, or a mental note, of all the techniques you find helpful. Be forward-looking and make plans for the future.

### Pacing after a Flare-Up

As the sensations ease off and you become confident that things are more stable, you can begin to start extending yourself again. Go very gently when you increase your activities. If your level of activity needs very critical monitoring, you could use the help of a countdown timer for basic activities such as sitting and walking, making very, very gradual increases in the times set. Take great care not to overdo things, and keep to the time you have allocated for yourself. This way *you* will stay in charge of the pain. Once you are feeling a little stronger, work through the Pacing Program in Unit 7. This will help you to lessen the chance of future flare-ups or setbacks and enable you to move through them more easily if they do occur.

Although you may not feel as though you want to exercise, you really do need to start moving in order to free up muscles that will probably have become stiff and sore. Moving makes us feel better about ourselves and often reduces the pain. Start a simple stretching program, even just for fingers and toes. The best form of exercise is the one you enjoy the most, and you may find it pleasurable to move to gentle music. Let the music flow around and over you, telling you how to move; just go with the rhythm. Keep as mobile as you can and space out your exercise throughout the day. If you notice any increase in pain at any time, stop what you are doing immediately.

As the flare-up comes to an end, take your time, especially if you are returning to work. Ideally, you could ease yourself back in with part-time work or working from home for a while. Sometimes, of course, when changes occur, you may have to accept that it is better not to use the "fast lane" of life at all. Accepting these kinds of changes can take time, but with the backup and support of the skills you can learn from the techniques in this book, you will have the knowledge and understanding to make the most of the hand you are dealt. Your spirit will fly even if your body cannot.

### *Affirmations for Flare-Ups*

Choose a few of the following affirmations for the different phases of a flare-up, or make up your own to suit your particular circumstances.

Repeat them often during the day. When we give ourselves positive thoughts, we change the way we feel about the flare-up and also the way in which we perceive the pain. Pain sensations diminish with the positive attitude we gain when we feel in control.

> *"I know what to do, I am in charge."*
> *"I accept the situation, I go with it. . . ."*
> *"I concentrate on what I can do."*
> *"There is plenty I can do to help myself."*
> *"I accept any help that is offered me."*
> *"There are plenty of others traveling this road: I am not alone."*
> *"Be calm, be peaceful, be patient."*
> *"It is easy for me to be patient."*
> *"I wait it out . . . there is plenty of time."*
> *"I am using this time as a learning period."*
> *"I am enjoying this break and the opportunity to practice some new skills."*
> *"Every day I get stronger and stronger."*
> *"I spend my time with enjoyable activities."*
> *"I enjoy finding new ways to cope."*
> *"I am open to new ideas."*
> *"I plan and pace myself through the day."*
> *"I take one step at a time."*
> *"I enjoy feeling my body move and become active again."*
> *"I take care of my body, I respect my body."*
> *"My body has served me well and I look after it."*
> *"I move through life with ease and joy."*

## Learning from Flare-Ups

Every crisis in life is an opportunity for personal growth. When we look back at our life with this in mind, we will be able to find that something good has come out of every difficult situation. We will have grown in some way personally, discovering aspects of ourselves or of life in general. These changes, which always please us, would probably not have been possible if we had not encountered and passed through those difficulties first. Flare-ups are a chance for us to make real progress in some way, either at a practical level, with some new way of handling the situation, or at a deeper, more spiritual level. Once the flare-up subsides, it is good to take a look back to see what we have learned.

*Make a note of the answers to these questions for future reference and to remind you of any action you may decide to take. Be totally honest with your answers in order to learn. The situation that caused the flare-up is in the past and cannot be changed, and now you can make good use of it.*

- *To avoid a flare-up occurring, could you have handled the situation that produced the flare-up differently?*
- *If so, how could you have handled it?*
- *Do you need to find any information or seek help from anyone else?*
- *What have you learned about what you can and cannot do easily?*
- *Can something in your routine be changed?*
- *Can you make some helpful changes in your environment?*
- *Did you lack confidence to say no to something when you knew it was too much for you?*
- *If you are going to make changes of any kind, what do you need to do?*
- *What have you learned about yourself during the flare-up?*
- *In which ways have your inner resources developed during this flare-up?*
- *Is there anything else you can learn from this flare-up?*
- *Is there anything else you can do?*
- *Is there anything you would like to do to help yourself generally or during any future flare-ups?*

*Give as full an answer as you can to the questions, making lists of ways to improve your lifestyle, if appropriate. Think hard about how you are going to make the changes that may be necessary. You may learn, for instance, that you need to slow down because you are attempting to do too much. To overcome a gen-*

*eral point like this, you need to think very carefully about how you are going to achieve your aim.*

*To support you during this questionnaire, choose from these affirmations or make up your own and repeat them often during the day when you come to the stage of doing this exercise.*

> *"This has been a great chance to learn more."*
> *"I acknowledge my achievements in adversity."*
> *"I acknowledge my personal growth."*
> *"I have done really well and it is wonderful to know that I am in control."*
> *"If this happens again, I am well prepared."*
> *"I enjoy continuing to learn and to grow."*
> *"All is well in my world."*

### *Praise and Congratulations*

Finally, it is important always to acknowledge your growth and to praise yourself for all your achievements along the way, no matter how small they seem. Acknowledge your achievements by recording them in your diary. Read them often and tell your friends and family about them. Don't be modest or minimize your achievements; we all do wonderfully well and do the best we can with the knowledge and understanding we currently have. Our ability to nourish and support ourselves increases daily as we gain more skills and become more and more in tune with our body's needs. We are learning to cope with something no one else can appreciate, and this deserves recognition. So tell yourself often that you love yourself, approve of yourself, and congratulate yourself on how well you are doing on what can be ultimately an uplifting and inspiring journey.

## SUMMARY

A flare-up can be a tremendous opportunity to learn more about yourself, to develop inner strengths, to learn how to cope with pain, and to appreciate the needs of your body. You will gain more awareness and have more understanding and knowledge available to you to help prevent flare-ups in the future. Don't stop learning when a flare-up is over; continue to find out as much as you can about yourself and your body, continue to practice basic skills such as relaxation, meditation, and natural diaphragmatic breathing. These techniques are beneficial to you whether or not you are in pain, and if you need them more intensively in the future, you will be well prepared.

In any flare-up situation in the future, remember the Flare-Up Action Plan, and know that you have the strategies and knowledge to support yourself toward a comforted, peaceful, and strengthened body, mind, and spirit.

### SUMMARY OF THE FLARE-UP ACTION PLAN

#### Step 1. "STOP"
*"I know what to do."*

#### Step 2. Diaphragmatic Breathing
*"I concentrate on my breathing."*
and
#### Affirmations
*"Relax—this will pass."*

#### Step 3. Select Next Strategy
Relaxation
Meditation
Visualization
Releasing Your Feelings
Encouraging Positive Emotions
Acceptance
Forgiveness
Pacing Yourself
Learning from the Flare-Up
Praise and Congratulations

# Continuing the Journey

A s you continue on your journey, you now have all you need to help you toward a healthier, more relaxed, peaceful, and enjoyable life than you may ever have thought possible. Always be open to new ideas and to learning about yourself and the world. Success with natural pain relief comes from knowing how to use the powers and strengths that are already within you.

Pack your life with joy, laughter, and fun to balance against the more difficult times and direct your attention toward plans and projects that inspire you with enthusiasm and enliven you with optimism. Plan your days and pace your activities so you don't overexert yourself, and make time for relaxation and exercise. Listen to and practice with the CD that accompanies this book, daily if you can. Remember to place your focus upon what you *can* do, and do not dwell upon what you can't do for the moment. Be kind to yourself; be true to yourself.

As you travel on, know that you are not alone. There are many hundreds of thousands on the path ahead, behind, and around you, passing through the same landscape with the same hills and mountains to climb—and sunny lowlands, peaceful rivers, and dappled woodlands to enjoy. Try to see the journey as a whole; if there is a hill to climb, there will surely be a sheltered valley to stroll through on the other side.

Reach out, reach out to others on the journey. It is through holding out our hand in friendship and love, giving hope and encouragement to others, that we transcend our own pain and lead a life of harmony and balance.

# Resources

## RECORDINGS AND BOOKS BY JAN SADLER

There are many recordings by Jan Sadler to complement this book. They include deeply peaceful and pain-relieving relaxation and visualization sessions and talks on natural pain relief and self-help pain management techniques, during which Jan gives many helpful ideas for reducing and coping with pain.

To find more information and to order downloads of recordings, CDs, or audiotapes, please visit www.painsupport.co.uk, Jan Sadler's Web site. The author recommends www.newworldmusic.com as a good source for relaxation music.

Other books by Jan Sadler are *Peaceful Sleep* and *The Five Feel-Good Factors*, both of which have accompanying recordings available as audiotape, CD, or download. Other recordings and booklets include *Pacing for Pain Relief* (used by many hospital pain management courses), *Relax and Release Your Pain,* and *Comfortable Sitting.*

### Online Support

**www.painsupport.co.uk**

If you have access to the Internet, you can log on to Jan Sadler's online support group, PainSUPPORT, where you can find advice, information on all aspects of self-help pain management, a lively discussion group, a regular newsletter (online and by e-mail), and a confidential Contact Club. Members of the Contact Club can get in touch with people who are in a similar situation for support and friendship.

# USEFUL ADDRESSES

## United States

### Pain Management Organizations

The American Chronic Pain
Association (ACPA)
PO Box 850
Rocklin, CA 95677-0850
800-533-3231
www.theacpa.org

American Pain Society (APS)
4700 W. Lake Ave.
Glenview, IL 60025
847-375-4715
www.ampainsoc.org

International Association for the Study
of Pain (IASP)
111 Queen Anne Ave. N., Suite 501
Seattle, WA 98109-4955
206-283-0311
www.iasp-pain.org

### Complementary Therapy Associations

American Academy of Medical
Acupuncture (AAMA)
4929 Wilshire Blvd., Suite 428
Los Angeles, CA 90010
323-937-5514
www.medicalacupuncture.org

American Chiropractic Association
1701 Clarendon Blvd.
Arlington, VA 22209
703-276-8800
www.amerchiro.org

American Herbalists Guild
141 Nob Hill Road
Cheshire, CT 06410
203-272-6731
www.americanherbalistsguild.com

American Holistic Medical Association
(AHMA)
PO Box 2016
Edmonds, WA 98020
425-967-0737
www.holisticmedicine.org

American Hypnosis Association
Hypnosis Motivation Institute
18607 Ventura Blvd., Suite 310
Tarzana, CA 91356-4158
818-758-2747
www.hypnosis.edu/aha

American Osteopathic Association
(AOA)
142 East Ontario St.
Chicago, IL 60611
800-621-1773
312-202-8000
www.osteopathic.org

American Physical Therapy Association
(APTA)
1111 North Fairfax St.
Alexandria, VA 22314-1488
800-999-2782
703-684-APTA (2782)
703-683-6748 (TDD)
www.apta.org

American Society for the Alexander
Technique (AmSAT)
PO Box 60008
Florence, MA 01062
800-473-0620
413-584-2359
www.alexandertech.com

Reflexology Association of America
(RAA)
4012 S. Rainbow Blvd. K-PMB# 585
Las Vegas, NV 89103-2059
702-871-9522
www.reflexology-usa.org

Rest Ministries, Inc.
PO Box 502928
San Diego, CA 92150
888-751-REST
858-486-4685
www.restministries.org

## Support for Specific Illnesses

**American Cancer Society (ACS)**
1599 Clifton Road, NE
Atlanta, GA 30329-4251
800-ACS-2345
866-228-4327 (TTY)
www.cancer.org

**American Fibromyalgia Syndrome
Association (AFSA)**
6380 E. Tanque Verde, Suite D
Tucson, AZ 85715
520-733-1570
www.afsafund.org

**Arthritis Foundation**
PO Box 7669
Atlanta, GA 30357-0669
800-568-4045
404-872-7100
404-965-7888
www.arthritis.org

**International Association for Chronic
Fatigue Syndrome (IACFS)**
27 North Wacker Drive, Suite 416
Chicago, IL 60606
847-258-7248
www.aacfs.org

**Spine-health.com**
123 W. Madison St., Suite 1450
Chicago, IL 60602
www.spine-health.com

**TNA (Trigeminal Neuralgia)**
925 Northwest 56th Terr., Suite C
Gainesville, FL 32605-6402
800-923-3608
352-331-7009
www.tna-support.org

**VZV Research Foundation (Shingles
and Post Herpetic Neuralgia)**
24 E. 64th St., 2nd Floor
New York, NY 10021
212-371-7280
www.vzvfoundation.org

## Other Helpful Contacts

**American Association of People with
Disabilities (AAPD)**
1629 K Street NW, Suite 503
Washington, DC 20006
800-840-8844 (V/TTY)
202-457-0046 (V/TTY)
www.aapd.com

## *United Kingdom*

### Pain Management Organizations

**Pain Association**
Cramond House
Cramond Glebe Road
EDINBURGH EH4 6NS
0800 783 6059
0131 312 7955
www.painassociation.com

**Pain Relief Foundation**
Clinical Sciences Centre
University Hospital Aintree
Lower Lane
LIVERPOOL L9 7AL
0151 529 5820
www.painrelieffoundation.org.uk

## Complementary Therapy Associations

**Association of Reflexologists**
5 Fore Street
TAUNTON
Somerset TA1 1HX
0870 567 332
For overseas callers: 01823 351010
www.reflexology.org/aor

**British Acupuncture Council**
63 Jeddo Road
LONDON W12 9HQ
020 8735 0400
www.acupuncture.org.uk

**British Chiropractic Association**
59 Castle Street
READING
Berkshire RG1 7SN
0118 950 5950
www.chiropractic-uk.co.uk

**British Holistic Medical Association**
PO Box 371
BRIDGWATER
Somerset TA6 9BG
0127 872 2000
www.bhma.org

**General Osteopathic Council**
176 Tower Bridge Road
LONDON SE1 3LU
020 7357 6655
www.osteopathy.org.uk

**Institute for Complementary Medicine (ICM)**
PO Box 194
LONDON SE16 7QZ
020 7237 5165
www.i-c-m.org.uk

**National Institute of Medical Herbalists (NIHM)**
Elm House
54 Mary Arches St.
EXETER EX4 3BA
01392 426 022
www.nimh.org.uk

**National Federation of Spiritual Healers**
Old Manor Farm Studio
Church Street
SUNBURY-ON-THAMES
Middlesex TW16 6RG
0845 123 2777
01932 783 164
www.region9-nfsh.co.uk
www.nfsh-region1.inuk.com

**National Register of Hypnotherapists and Psychotherapists (NRHP)**
Suite B
12 Cross St.
NELSON
Lancs BB9 7EN
01282 716 839
www.nrhp.co.uk

**The Society of Homeopaths**
11 Brookfield
Duncan Close, Moulton Park
NORTHAMPTON NN3 6WL
0845 450 6611
www.homeopathy-soh.org

**The Society of Teachers of the Alexander Technique (STAT)**
Linton House, 1st Floor
39-51 Highgate Road
LONDON NW5 1RS
0845 230 7828
www.stat.org.uk

## Support for Specific Illnesses

**Arthritis Care**
18 Stephenson Way
LONDON NW1 2HD
Helpline: 0808 800 4050
020 7380 6500
www.arthritiscare.org.uk

**BackCare (formerly National Back Pain Association)**
16 Elmtree Road
TEDDINGTON
Middlesex TW11 8ST
Helpline: 0845 130 2704
44 20 8977 5474
www.backcare.org/uk

**The Bristol Cancer Help Centre**
Grove House
Cornwallis Grove
BRISTOL BS8 4PG
Helpline: 0845 123 2310
0117 980 9500
www.bristolcancerhelp.org

**Cancerbackup**
3 Bath Place
Rivington Street
LONDON EC2A 3JR
Helpline: 0808 800 1234
www.cancerbackup.org

**Fibromyalgia Association UK**
PO Box 206
STOURBRIDGE
West Midlands DY9 8YL
0870 752 5118
www.fibromyalgia-associationuk.org

## Other Helpful Contacts

**Disabled Living Foundation**
380-384 Harrow Road
LONDON W9 2HU
Helpline: 0845 130 9177
020 7289 6111
www.dlf.org.uk

**NHS Direct, UK**
24-hour helpline: 0845 4647
www.nhsdirect.nhs.uk

**NHS Help for Health Trust, UK**
0800 66 55 44
*Health information service: information available about any health matter, leaflets sent, books lent. Details of hospital services, including Pain Management Clinics*

**Remap**
D9 Chaucer Business Park
KEMSING TN15 6YU
0845 130 0456
www.remap.org.uk
*A charity that makes specialized equipment for disabled people to help with daily living*

## Australia

**Australian Natural Therapists
Association (ANTA)**
PO Box 657
Maroochydore QLD 4558
1800 817 577
07 5409 8222
www.anta.com.au

**Australian Pain Society**
Dc Conferences Pty Ltd
Suite 1, ground floor
26 Ridge St.
North Sydney NSW 2060
02 9954 4400
www.apsoc.org.au

**National Herbalists Association of
Australia (NHAA)**
PO Box 45
Concord West NSW 2138
02 8765 0071
www.nhaa.org.au

## Canada

**Chronic Pain Association of Canada
(CPAC)**
PO Box 66017
Heritage Postal Station
#130 2323-111 St.
Edmonton, AB T6J 6T4
780-482-6727
www.chronicpaincanada.com

**Ontario Herbalists Association**
RR #1
Port Burwell, ON N0J 1T0
877-OHA-HERB
416-236-0090
www.herbalists.on.ca

**West Coast Homeopathic Society**
#101-10001 West Broadway, Unit 120
Vancouver, BC V6H 4E4
604-803-9242
www.wchs.info/index.htm

## France

**Association Française de Chiropratique**
24, rue de Monttessuy
75007 Paris
www.chiropratique.org

**Société Medical de Biothérapie
(Homeopathy)**
62, rue Beaubourg
75003 Paris

## New Zealand

**Herb Federation of New Zealand**
PO Box 42
Katikati 3063
www.herbs.org.nz

**New Zealand Pain Society**
PO Box 5303
Wellington
www.nzps.org.nz

**New Zealand Register of
Acupuncturists Inc.**
PO Box 9950
Wellington 6001
04 476 4866
www.acupuncture.org.nz

**Osteopathic Society of New Zealand
(OSNZ)**
PO Box 647
Rangiora
03 313 5086
www.osnz.org

# Recommended Books

## UNIT 1: THE POWER OF DEEP RELAXATION

Benson, Herbert, with Miriam Z. Klipper. *The Relaxation Response.* Exp. and rev. ed. New York: Quill, 2001.

Craze, Richard. *Teach Yourself Relaxation.* 2nd ed. New York: McGraw-Hill, 2005.

Davis, Martha, Elizabeth Eshelman Robbins, and Matthew McKay. *The Relaxation and Stress Reduction Workbook.* 5th ed. Oakland, Calif.: New Harbinger, 2000.

Madders, Jane. *Stress and Relaxation.* New York: Arco Publishing, 1993

Weekes, Claire. *Self Help for Your Nerves.* 3rd ed. New York: HarperCollins, 2000.

Wilson, Paul. *Instant Calm.* New York: Plume Books, 1995.

## UNIT 2: WHAT ARE YOU TELLING YOURSELF?

Bandler, Richard, and John Grinder. *Frogs into Princes: Neuro Linguistic Programming.* Moab, Utah: Real People Press, 1979.

Hay, Louise. *You Can Heal Your Life.* Santa Monica, Calif.: Hay House, 1987.

Jeffers, Susan. *Feel the Fear and Do It Anyway.* Rev. ed. New York: MJF Books, 2006.

McWilliams, Peter. *You Can't Afford the Luxury of a Negative Thought.* Rev. ed. Los Angeles: Prelude Press, 1995.

## UNIT 3: BUILDING SELF-ESTEEM AND A POSITIVE ATTITUDE

Broome, Annabel, and Helen Jellicoe. *Living with Your Pain.* Oxford, UK: Taylor & Francis Books, 1987.

Peiffer, Vera. *Positive Thinking.* Rockport, Mass.: Element Books, 1994.

Proto, Louis. *Self-Healing: Use Your Mind to Heal Your Body.* York Beach, Maine: Weiser, 1991.

Roger, John, and Peter McWilliams. *Do It!* New York: HarperCollins, 1992, 2001.

## UNIT 4: PICTURES IN YOUR MIND

Gawain, Shakti. *Creative Visualization*. Navato, Calif.: New World Library, 2002.

Gawler, Ian. *The Creative Power of Imagery*. South Yarra, Australia: Michelle Anderson Publishing, 1998.

Simonton, Carl O., Stephanie Matthews-Simonton, and James L. Creighton. *Getting Well Again*. New York: Bantam Books, 1992.

## UNIT 5: DEALING WITH YOUR FEELINGS

Blackburn, Ivy. *Coping with Depression*. Edinburgh: Chambers Harrap, 1987.

Nash, Wanda. *At Ease with Stress*. Mystic, Conn.: Twenty-Third Publications, 1991.

Roet, Brian. *A Safer Place to Cry*. London: Century Hutchinson, 1989.

Trickett, Shirley. *Coping with Anxiety and Depression*. 2nd ed. London: Sheldon Press, 1996.

## UNIT 6: FINDING THE STILLNESS WITHIN

Bancroft, Anne. *The Spiritual Journey*. Rockport, Mass.: Element, 1991.

Hewitt, James. *Meditation*. London: Teach Yourself, 1994.

Kabat-Zinn, Jon. *Full Catastrophe Living*. Reissue. New York: Delta, 2005.

LeShan, Lawrence. *How to Meditate*. Boston: Little, Brown, 1999.

Macbeth, Jessica. *Moon Over Water*. Rev. ed. Lithia Springs, Ga.: New Leaf, 2002.

Nhat Hanh, Thich. *Be Still and Know*. New York: Riverhead Trade, 1996.

## UNIT 7: PACING AND PLANNING YOUR ACTIVITIES

Parker, Helen, and Chris J. Main. *Living with Back Pain*. New York: Manchester University Press, 1990.

Wheeler, Eugenie G. *Living Creatively with Chronic Illness*. Ventura, Calif.: Pathfinder, 1989.

## UNIT 8: ENJOYING YOURSELF

Baum, Glenda. *Aquarobics*. London: Arrow, 1991.

Capaccione, Lucia. *Recovery of Your Inner Child*. New York: Simon & Schuster, 1991.

Csikszentmihalyi, Mihaly. *Flow: The Psychology of Optimal Experience*. New York: Harper, 1991.

Edwards, Betty. *The New Drawing on the Right Side of the Brain*. Rev. and exp. ed. New York: Tarcher/Putnam, 1999.

Hoffmann, David. *The New Holistic Herbal*. Rockport, Mass.: Element, 1990.

Lewith, George, and Sandra Horn. *Drug Free Pain Relief* (TENS information). New York: Thorsons, 1987.

Maxwell-Hudson, Clare. *The Complete Book of Massage*. London: Dorling Kindersley, 1988.

Trickett, Shirley. *Coming off Tranquilizers*. 2nd ed. New York: Thorsons, 1994.

## UNIT 9: FLARE-UP ACTION PLAN

Goldhawk, Tessa. *A Rose to a Sick Friend*. Santa Rosa, Calif.: Atrium Publishers Group, 1989.

LeMaistre, Joann. *Beyond Rage*. Rev. and exp. ed. Oak Park, Ill.: Alpine Guild, 1993.

Manning, Matthew. *Matthew Manning's Guide to Self Healing*. New York: Harper-Collins, 1989.

Wells, Chris, and Graham Nown. *The Pain Relief Handbook*. Richmond Hill, Ontario: Firefly Books, 1998.

## OTHER RECOMMENDED BOOKS

Catalano, Ellen Mohr, and Kimeron Hardin. *The Chronic Pain Control Workbook*. New York: MJF Books, 1997.

Chopra, Deepak. *Quantum Healing*. New York: Bantam Books, 1989.

Cousins, Norman. *Anatomy of an Illness as Perceived by the Patient*. Rep. ed. New York: Norton, 2005.

Drake, Jonathan. *The Alexander Technique in Everyday Life*. New York: Thorsons, 1996.

———. *Body Knowhow* (Alexander Technique). New York: HarperCollins, 1992.

Hall, Hamilton. *Be Your Own Back Doctor*. New York: HarperCollins, 1983.

Holford, Patrick, and Jennifer Meek. *Boost Your Immune System*. London: Piatkus, 1998.

Key, Sarah. *Back in Action*. London: Vermilion, 2001.

Jayson, Malcolm I. V. *Back Pain: The Facts*. New York: Oxford University Press, 1995.

Klein, Arthur C., and Dava Sobel. *Backache: What Exercises Work*. New York: St. Martin's, 1996.

McTaggart, Lynne. *What Doctors Don't Tell You*. Rep. ed. New York: HarperCollins, 2005.

Shone, Neville. *Coping Successfully with Pain*. 2nd ed. London: Sheldon Press, 2003.

Siegel, Bernie. *Love, Medicine and Miracles*. New York: HarperPerennial, 1990.

Turner, Roger Newman. *Banish Back Pain*. New York: HarperCollins, 1996.

Wall, Patrick. *Pain: The Science of Suffering*. New York: Columbia University Press, 2000.

Wall, Patrick, and Mervyn Jones. *Defeating Pain*. New York: Plenum Press, 1991.

Wells, Chris. *In Pain?* London: Century Hutchinson, 1993.

White, Augustus A. *Your Aching Back: A Doctor's Guide to Relief*. New York: Fireside, 1990.

Young, Jacqueline. *Acupressure Step by Step*. New York: Thorsons, 1998.

# Index

# Books of Related Interest

**THE ACUPUNCTURE TREATMENT OF PAIN**
*Safe and Effective Methods for Using Acupuncture in Pain Relief*
Leon Chaitow, D.O., N.D.

**ACUPRESSURE TECHNIQUES**
*A Self-Help Guide*
Julian Kenyon, M.D.

**TRIGGER POINT SELF-CARE MANUAL**
*For Pain-Free Movement*
Donna Finando, L.Ac., L.M.T.

**TRIGGER POINT THERAPY FOR MYOFASCIAL PAIN**
*The Practice of Informed Touch*
Donna Finando, L.Ac., L.M.T., and
Steven Finando, Ph.D., L.Ac.

**BUDDHIST HEALING TOUCH**
*A Self-Care Program for Pain Relief and Wellness*
Ming-Sun Yen, M.D., Joseph Chiang, M.D.,
and Myrna Louison Chen

**THE REFLEXOLOGY ATLAS**
Bernard C. Kolster, M.D., and Astrid Waskowiak, M.D.

**THE REFLEXOLOGY MANUAL**
*An Easy-to-Use Illustrated Guide to
the Healing Zones of the Hands and Feet*
Pauline Wills

**LUPUS**
*Alternative Therapies That Work*
Sharon Moore

Inner Traditions • Bear & Company
P.O. Box 388
Rochester, VT 05767
1-800-246-8648
www.InnerTraditions.com

Or contact your local bookseller